About the book

Hello, and welcome to my book!

I am Noorali Bharwani. This book is about life, my life. A life lived in four continents. A life in which I met many interesting people, experienced many interesting things and visited many interesting places. That makes for interesting stories.

The stories are about my family and friends, about kindness and caring, about laughter and happiness, about good health and bad health, about success and disappointments, about peace and sufferings and about religion and nirvana.

I know you will relate to many of these stories and find them compelling, emotional and humorous. So, go for it!

My website:
www.nbharwani.com

Note for Librarians: A cataloguing record for this book is available from Library and Archives Canada at www.collectionscanada.ca/amicus/index-e.html
ISBN 1-4120-9156-X

Printed in Victoria, BC, Canada. Printed on paper with minimum 30% recycled fibre. Trafford's print shop runs on "green energy" from solar, wind and other environmentally-friendly power sources.

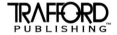

Offices in Canada, USA, Ireland and UK

Book sales for North America and international:
Trafford Publishing, 6E–2333 Government St.,
Victoria, BC V8T 4P4 CANADA
phone 250 383 6864 (toll-free 1 888 232 4444)
fax 250 383 6804; email to orders@trafford.com
Book sales in Europe:
Trafford Publishing (UK) Limited, 9 Park End Street, 2nd Floor
Oxford, UK OX1 1HH UNITED KINGDOM
phone +44 (0)1865 722 113 (local rate 0845 230 9601)
facsimile +44 (0)1865 722 868; info.uk@trafford.com
Order online at:
trafford.com/06-0910

10 9 8 7 6 5 4 3

Dr. Noorali Bharwani

A Doctor's Journey

an emotional
and humorous look at life
through the eyes of a doctor

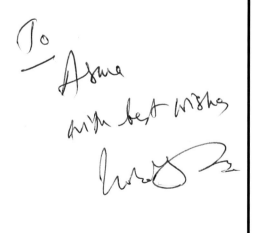

TRAFFORD
PUBLISHING™

Cover page photograph and concept by
Hussein Bharwani

Edited by
Alisha Sims
Leah Prestayko
Dennis van Westerborg

Published by
Noorali Bharwani Professional Corporation
821A-5th Street SW
Medicine Hat, Alberta, T1A 4H7
Canada
Website: *www.nbharwani.com*

Disclaimer

Permission to reprint

Cartoons in Chapters 7, 13 and 19 printed with the permission of Mr. Rick Campbell, editor, *The Medical Post*

Cartoons in Chapters 2, 22 and 23 printed with the permission of Mr. Simon Hally, editor, *Stitches, The Journal of Medical Humour.*

Photograph in "About the Author" printed with the permission of Mr. Tom Trombley, Impact Studios, Medicine Hat, Alberta.

Newspaper clippings from the *Medicine Hat News* printed with the permission of Mr. Alan Poirier, managing editor, the *Medicine Hat News*.

Contents

About the author

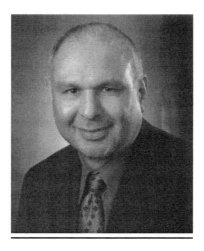

Dr. Noorali Bharwani was born and raised in Tanzania and has lived in India, Britain and Canada.

After finishing high school in Tanzania, Noorali went to India for higher education. Noorali is a graduate of the Prince of Wales Medical College, University of Patna in Patna, India. He received his surgical training in Britain and Canada. He is a Member of the Royal College of Surgeons of England, Licentiate of the Royal College of Physicians of London, Fellow of the Royal College of Surgeons of Glasgow, Fellow of the Royal College of Surgeons of Edinburgh, Fellow of the Royal College of Physicians and Surgeons of Canada, Fellow of the American College of Surgeons and Licentiate of the Medical Council of Canada.

In 1979, Noorali started work in Canada as a Research Fellow of the National Cancer Institute of Canada and as a Scientific and Research Associate of the Southern Alberta Cancer Clinic in Calgary, Alberta. He did his Surgical Residency Program in Edmonton. He

Dr. Noorali Bharwani

has worked as a Specialist in General Surgery in Medicine Hat since 1985. He was Regional Chief of Staff for the Palliser Health Region in south-eastern Alberta for about four years. In the past he has been a volunteer, a board member, vice-president, president and provincial board member for the Medicine Hat branch of the Canadian Cancer Society. He writes a regular health and wellness column for the *Medicine Hat News* and the *Oyen Echo*. He has written articles for *The Medical Post* as well and has published articles in scientific journals.

Noorali is a family man and enjoys his time with his wife and two children. He enjoys writing, biking, walking, downhill skiing (green runs only), swimming (not in the deep end), golfing (with a slice) and reading newspapers and magazines. And he enjoys his work as a surgeon.

Dedicated to

My wife, Sabiya, who has stood by me for many years, keeping the family together while I was spending long hours in the operating room, attending meetings, recruiting doctors or snoring the night away after inhaling all the gases in the surgical suites.

My children, Hussein and Alia, who are so precious and kind, whose gentle critique keeps me challenged in all walks of life.

My parents, brothers and sisters, who were very patient and helped me during my many university years away from home, when I moved from one country to another and during some turbulent times in my life.

My patients and readers of my newspaper column. Without them this book would not have been possible.

My teachers in Tanzania, India, Britain and Canada, who taught me many wonderful things and treated me like their son or friend.

Numerous families in these countries who took care of me during my high school, college and university days when I was away from home, sometimes lonely and hungry.

And the people of Medicine Hat for making us feel at home.

Quotes

I quote others in order to better express myself.
~ Michel de Montaigne (1533-1592)

The greatest thing in the world is to know how to be oneself.
~ Michel de Montaigne (1533-1592)

A man travels the world in search of what he needs and returns home to find it.
~ George Moore (1852-1933)

Change is what keeps us fresh and innovative. Change is what keeps us from getting stale. Change is what keeps us young.
~ Rick Pitino in *"Success Is A Choice"*

One can never consent to creep when one feels an impulse to soar.
~ Helen Keller (1880-1968)

Life has no meaning; you have to bring your own.
~ Dennis van Westerborg in *"Images and Reflections"*

Acknowledgements

My desire, during my surgical training years and after, was to write a text book of surgery. A book that would be simple to read, easy to understand and be humorous. But that project hasn't started yet. Instead, I wrote a book about life, religion and medicine as I saw it. I have been a freelance newspaper columnist since 1998. Writing a book has been a different but an exciting experience. Since this was my first time, I went around knocking at many doors, looking for advice and encouragement.

I soon realized how lucky I was to have friends who have written books or are in newspaper publishing business. When I asked for help and favours, none of them turned me down. They encouraged me and answered my questions. Some of them reviewed and edited the manuscript and suggested creative changes and improvements. They monitored my progress. They kept me going. Gordon Wright and Alisha Sims wrote a foreword and an introduction respectively. What a wonderful icing on the cake. I am one lucky person to have friends like these.

To all of them I owe more than a thank you for their truly genuine friendship, for their time and patience and for their kindness and generosity:

Gordon Wright, editor of daily newspapers in Canada
Martin and Marian Jerry, authors of *Sutras of the Inner Teacher*
Dennis van Westerborg, author of *Images and Reflections*
Alan Poirier, managing editor, the *Medicine Hat News*
Leah Prestayko, associate editor, the *Medicine Hat News*
Alisha Sims, copy editor, the *Medicine Hat News*
Michael Mirolla, editor, award-winning fiction writer and creative writing tutor
Joyce White, author and editor

Dr. Noorali Bharwani

Barbara Sibbald, author and medical journalist
Jana Pruden, author of *Robin Killer* and journalist
Rick Campbell, editor, *The Medical Post,* for permission to reprint
cartoons in Chapters 7, 13 and 19
Simon Hally, editor, *Stitches, The Journal of Medical Humour,* for
permission to reprint cartoons in Chapters 2, 22 and 23
and
Sabiya, Hussein and Alia Bharwani, my very patient family
Thank you all.

Foreword

by Gordon Wright

In our global village, Noorali Bharwani is a great neighbour. This emerging author is an accomplished physician, a caring humanitarian and a fine citizen of the world who understands the true value of family and friendships.

If you have not met him face-to-face, you will soon know his character as you page through this book. Whether you share the same postal code, the same city, country, or planet, you will find him to be a true friend and neighbour.

I have learned this from many a positive experience.

When needed, Noorali is there for you with a positive outlook. He is a willing helper. He is a builder. He is a contributor. He is a man of medicine. He is a spiritual leader in his own way. And, when appropriate, he is a sympathetic counselor with sage advice.

He is willing to share. Sharing is what this book is about.

A surgeon by profession, he has been very well educated on a few vastly different continents. He is well travelled – life has moved him from the lush shores of Lake Victoria, Tanzania to the desert of Medicine Hat, Alberta. A son, a husband, a father and a multi-level in-law, he shares the collective wisdom of an extensive extended family.

It is easy to get to know Noorali and make friends. He greets you with a warm handshake, a relaxed demeanor and a friendly grin. I've also learned to check for the telltale sparkle in his eyes. Often, the light that shines bright indicates there is a provocative idea percolating in his mind. The idea will always be worth exploring.

Of course, this book started out in the gleam of his eyes. But it is also a product of his work ethic and determination. He gets results. The wisdom and wit collected on these pages is worth sharing. Read on. Get to know Noorali, his family and friends. And, when you find something worth savouring, share it with other friends or neighbours in our global village. Let them know where you read it. Enjoy.

— Gord Wright, editor of daily newspapers in Canada

Introduction

by Alisha Sims

"What can I do for you today?"

How many times have we had a physician walk into the examination room and ask us that question? But in the case of Dr. Noorali Bharwani it's not a matter of *what* he can do for his patients, it's what he's *done* for his patients.

In addition to running a successful general surgical practice in Medicine Hat, Alberta, the Tanzanian-born physician has been involved in the administrative aspect of health care as well. In 1997, Noorali took on the job of Regional Chief of Medical Staff (RCOS) for the Palliser Health Authority. The administrative position calls for being a combination of a physician manager and a liaison officer between the health authority and the physicians. In other words, he was a sort of messenger who was liable to be shot from both sides if things didn't go right.

He had his share of critics. They said the job would be more stressful than working round the clock as a surgeon. They thought he was too kind, too soft and too emotional to tackle difficult problems and handle some difficult physicians. Even though he can have an intimidating physical presence, being 6'2" tall, his soft-spoken nature, quiet demeanour and occasional aloofness were interpreted as his weakness.

Don't be fooled though. As a surgeon he is a perfectionist and a fixer of problems.

Noorali started his general surgical practice in Medicine Hat, Alberta in 1985. Since then he has touched the lives of almost every family in the region and surrounding areas through his surgical expertise, through his newspaper columns on health and wellness and through his health related educational "info-mercials" on a Medicine Hat television station.

Noorali has handled many difficult surgical cases and has made tough decisions in many life threatening situations. So he is no stranger to making tough decisions. He looks back at his surgical career with great satisfaction and continues to provide his service to the people of the region.

Noorali is happy with his record as a physician-administrator as well. He was in that position for close to four years. His biggest contributions to the well being of the physicians and the people of Palliser health region can be summarized as follows:

He encouraged aggressive regional recruitment program for new family physicians and specialists. As a result the health authority recruited about one physician a month in the region.

He initiated many projects to improve the working environment for the physicians in Medicine Hat and rural areas of Oyen, Bassano, Brooks and Bow Island.

He encouraged improvement in the organizational structure and patient safety and risk management committees of the medical staff.

He pushed for improved communication and interaction between the physicians, the senior administration and the regional health board members by organizing joint meetings, social functions and a monthly newsletter (*The Way I See It—from the Regional Chief of Staff*).

Of course, many other things were done, and many problems and crisis were faced and taken care of by Noorali, but these are among the most noteworthy administrative work.

Noorali loves a good challenge and wishes he can fix everything and make it right. But in life one has to accept certain things will never change. As a self-described obsessive, compulsive perfectionist surgeon, Noorali admits having trouble accepting that.

But that's an integral part of who Noorali is—a fixer. From his days spent as a young man writing letters to the editor about the politics of the day to writing newspaper columns today promoting general health, Noorali looks to make the world we live in a better place. And, really, in the grand scheme of things, isn't that the ultimate prescription to cure what ails mankind?

– Alisha Sims
(Alisha is a copy editor at the Medicine Hat News.
She was the paper's acting associate editor from 2004-05).

1

A pilgrim's progress

Musoma to Medicine Hat

The stature of a man is not measured in how far he has gone, but in knowing the distance he has come from.
~ Unknown Author

I was born in Musoma, Tanzania, on August 25, 1945. My mom was 26 years old and my dad was 33. My mom had a difficult labour because I was a breech baby. She said I weighed seven pounds. I was heavier than my siblings, who were about six pounds. I was delivered at home by a traditional, unqualified but experienced midwife.

I was the sixth child in my family. Oldest was my sister Gulshan, next was my sister Zarin, then my sister Gulzar who died at the age of five from jaundice, then my brother Esmail and then my sister Shahsultan (Shully). After my birth, my mother bore two more children, both boys, Mansur and Anil.

Musoma is in Tanganyika which is the mainland portion of what later became Tanzania. In the late 19th century, Tanganyika was under German occupation. The town of Musoma was created by the Germans as a fortification point. The name Musoma means promontory or peninsula and the name is derived from a local dialect.

After the First World War, Tanganyika was administered by Britain under the League of Nations mandate and later as a United Nations trust territory.

In 1961, I was 15 years old when Tanganyika became an independent nation. I was a keen reader of newspapers and daily listener to the BBC World Service. I was not a political activist but took a keen interest in following the events leading to independence. The neighbouring countries of Kenya and Uganda went through the same process but their paths were more complicated due to the presence of multiple political factions.

When I was growing up, Musoma was a relatively small town in the Mara region. The population of Musoma and the Mara region has grown from half a million in the 1960s to approximately 1.5 million today.

I lived in Musoma until I was 14 and finished Grade 9. I studied at the Aga Khan School. School was fun and after school hours there were many sporting activities to take part in. I played all kinds of sports including volleyball, badminton, field hockey, soccer, tennis and cricket.

Sometimes after school we had Boy Scout meetings, band practice or I would go to my dad's shop and help him. Like most traders of Asian origin in East Africa, my dad was a general merchant. His specialty was selling clothes and fabrics geared to local needs. From time to time he also tried his hand at selling other merchandise such as bicycles, timber and ghee (a clarified semi-solid butter used especially in Indian cooking). He had a large family to feed and educate. He worked very hard. At one time he owned three shops, which kept my mom, two older sisters and brother busy.

I was brought up in a very religious family. Attending to daily prayers was almost mandatory. In the evenings, we had to be home by six or so to shower, get ready and go to the local prayer hall called *jamatkhana*. My mom and dad were very involved in community service in various capacities. For more than 30 years, my dad and mom presided over many congregations (*majalis*) in *jamatkhanas*.

One of the congregations met at four in the morning to meditate and pray. I remember, as a child, I would accompany my dad to go to *jamatkhana* to meditate. There was no electricity. We walked in the darkness of the night with a small kerosene lamp, not knowing what was ahead of us. I used to be scared of the barking dogs, and afraid of being attacked by thieves and robbers. Luckily, nothing happened.

I like to sit in meditation. I have been brought up with the idea that the best time to meditate is at four in the morning. It is very peaceful. Your previous day's worries are gone and you have not started your new day yet. Your mind and body is rested and has the ability to concentrate. Unfortunately I have not kept up with this. I have been too busy doing other worldly things, such as working around the clock as a surgeon and raising a family. But the sense of spirituality descends on you as you get older. I am getting to that point in my life.

Growing up in a small town like Musoma was fun. Biking was my passion. On weekends I would spend long hours riding around the town on my bike. I would go to the post office to collect mail. On Sundays I would go to Musoma Pier on Lake Victoria to buy bunches of bananas, which would arrive from Uganda by boat. I would carry the bananas, sometimes on the steering wheel as well as on the back rack of my bike, and take them home, which was a two-kilometer ride.

My bicycle antics made me fall several times. I have a few scars on my body, especially on my shins, from cuts and bruises. In addition to biking, we used to walk a lot. My dad and mom enjoyed walking. We did not own a car, so if we wanted to go somewhere we either walked or biked.

Grade 9 was as far as I could study in Musoma. There was no secondary school. So in 1960, at the age of 14, I had to go to a boarding school in Dar-es-Salaam, the capital city of Tanzania. From Musoma, I travelled by boat overnight to Mwanza, and then rode a train to Dar-es-Salaam. The train journey was two-and-a-half days. It was slow, dusty and hot.

Dar-es-Salaam had a population of about 350,000. The population has now risen to 2.5 million. Dar-es-Salaam is an Arabic word meaning "haven of peace." In the late 1800s, the city was ruled by the Arabs. Then came the Germans and the British. Life in Dar-es-Salaam revolves around the huge harbour on the Indian Ocean.

I studied at the Aga Khan Boys' School in Dar-es-Salaam, for two years and completed Grade 10 and 11. I used to go home every three months during the school holidays. Each time I found the journey very long and annoying, but it was good to get away from the boarding school and the terrible food served there. Going home meant being spoiled by my mom.

By this time economic conditions in Musoma were becoming difficult. My father needed a change so he moved the family to Mwanza, another Lake Victoria town, which is bigger than Musoma. Mwanza had a secondary school, Chopra Secondary School. So, in 1962, at the age of 17, I left the boarding school in Dar-es-Salaam to finish Grade 12 in Mwanza.

Mwanza had a population of about one million. Now the population is about 2.6 million. The city of Mwanza is the major Tanzanian port on Lake Victoria and a major centre of economic importance in the region.

After one year in Mwanza, it was time to move again. I wanted to become a doctor. There was no medical school in East Africa except for one in Uganda, which had just started accepting students. I had to go overseas to pursue further studies. The two most popular places to go were the United Kingdom and India. India was more affordable so I applied to Wadia College in Poona and was accepted to study science. Poona, also known as Pune, is located in the western Indian state of Maharashtra.

While waiting to attend college in India, I took up a job as a temporary teacher for six months at the Aga Khan Primary School in Mwanza. That was good experience. Besides the headmaster, I was the only other male teacher amongst all the female teachers. There was a trend in East Africa that saw more female teachers in primary schools than in secondary schools.

In 1963, I proceeded to Poona to study science and find a spot in a medical school. The journey from Tanzania to India was a slow process by train and boat. Air travel was expensive and we could not afford it. From Mwanza, I travelled by train to Dar-es-Salaam which was a two-and-a-half-day journey. I would stay in Dar-es-Salaam for a night or two and then take a ship to go to Bombay, now called Mumbai.

In Dar-es-Salaam, I was always taken care of by the family of Hassanali Kassum Sunderji. They were a very caring, kind and generous family and I knew them from my days in the boarding school when they used to look after several boarders on the weekends. As fate would have it, many years later I married their youngest daughter, Sabiya.

From Dar-es-Salaam the ship would navigate through the Indian Ocean and make a five-hour stop in Zanzibar and then dock for three nights in Mombasa, Kenya. From Mombasa it was a seven-day journey to Bombay with brief stopovers at Seychelles Island or Karachi in Pakistan. From Mwanza to Bombay was a two-week journey. Like the majority of the East African students studying in India, I could not afford to fly and travelled by boat. We travelled in the third-class section. This was the cheapest way to go to India. The bunks in the third-class section were crowded, hot and humid. It was difficult to sleep. Sometimes we slept on the deck to get some fresh air, but we would be showered with salty mist as the big waves hit the ship.

In the summer months, the Indian Ocean was rough. Moving around on the ship's deck was not always easy. The waves would rock the boat from side to side. Aluminum food trays, known as thali, on aluminum tables would slide from one end to the other. If you were not fast enough to stop the slide then your food would end up on the floor. Many passengers were sea sick. Combined with the fact that the food was terrible and nausea and vomiting made eating almost impossible, especially after watching people throw up right in front of you.

I studied science for a year in Poona. Poona is a beautiful city. I had two great local friends, Bhagwan Sadarangani and Harry Moorjani. We used to bike a lot. After I left India, I lost touch with Bhagwan and Harry. I heard Bhagwan had moved to the U.S. after he finished medical school in India. One day, in 2005, I was sitting in my office and out of curiosity I typed Bhagwan's name on the Google Internet search engine. His name, address and phone number appeared on the screen. He was in New York.

I picked up the phone and called him. I found out he was a general surgeon as well. We talked for half an hour or so. After 40 years, we established contact again. We exchanged family pictures and plan to meet in the near future. He told me he was in touch with Harry, who is still in Poona. I really enjoyed my year in Poona. We used to make frequent weekend trips to Bombay via a three-hour express train. Bombay is a fun city as well.

After a year of science in Poona, I was nominated by the Government of India to study medicine at the Prince of Wales Medical College (also known as Patna Medical College) in Patna, Bihar. Patna had a program which integrated one-year of pre-medicine.

The journey from Poona to Bombay wasn't bad. I travelled by train, third class again. At approximately 1 a.m. I had to take the train from Bombay to Allahabad – a 24-hour journey. Then the nightmare started. When I arrived in Allahabad the following night, I had to get my luggage out, change platforms and then take a train to Patna. The train going to Patna had no room, and I had too much luggage. A porter helped me shove my entire luggage near the door of one of the compartments. I had to sit on my luggage all night right at the door of the train compartment. I don't know how I did it. When I think of it now, I think it was insane. But that is how life is in one of the most populated countries in the world. Trains and buses are always overcrowded.

I arrived at Patna station at around six in the morning. There was nobody at the station so I waited till about at 8 a.m. I was able to find a rickshaw to take me to the medical college residence. That was in 1964. I was only 19 years old! I was in a totally unfamiliar country. My parents were worried about me, but I was not scared because I was very excited to be accepted in a medical school. I was happy to be in Patna. Within a year, I was accepted in the bursary program of His Highness the Aga Khan Education Board for Tanzania. That meant my medical education in Patna was financed by the education board. This came as a great relief as my parents had to save to finance the education for other members of the family.

Patna was a very crowded and dirty city. I don't know if much has changed in the last 30 to 40 years. Politically, the State of Bihar was very unstable. The state government would fall every six months. The local politicians would change allegiance to their parties frequently. There was a significant tension based on religion and caste. I have witnessed few political and religious riots. I was there when India and Pakistan went to war and saw the separation of East Pakistan as an independent nation of Bangladesh.

I had some good friends in Patna. There were at least five local families who took interest in my welfare. There were many foreign students from different parts of the world. We had our own association and cultural activities. We mixed well with the local population. During holidays, I visited different parts of India, including the Taj Mahal. I also made a trip to Nepal for a couple of days. The only thing I remember about Kathmandu is it rained non-stop for the two days I was there and the hotel room had a leaky roof!

Mansur, my younger brother, also joined me in Patna. He graduated from the Patna University with First Class honours in Statistics.

After my internship, I left Patna for the United Kingdom. The plan was to be a surgeon. I had to wait for a few months in London before I could finalize my licensing procedure with the General Medical Council. During those months I took up a job as a stock boy at one of the large grocery stores. It wasn't a very pleasant experience and I did not last there more than a couple of weeks.

Once I got my licence to practice in the U.K. I had to find a position where I could spend a month for assessment of my clinical skills. A very kind elderly surgeon accepted me at the London Jewish Hospital. For the surgical trainees, there was no structured residency program in the U.K. Every six to 12 months we had to move from one hospital to another. That meant loading my car and moving to the next city.

I started my surgical training in southern England in Dartford, Kent. I stayed in Dartford for close to three years and rotated between two hospitals. I trained in trauma, orthopedics and general surgery. Then I moved to London and worked six months at the Hospital for Sick Children on Great Ormond Street, training in pediatric cardio-thoracic surgery. My next move was to Middlesborough, in northern England near New Castle upon Tyne. I lived there for 18 months and trained in General Surgery and Neurosurgery. From there I went to London again to train at the Hammersmith Hospital in Urology and Renal Transplantation. My last move was to Margate, Kent, where I worked for just over six months in general surgery before I moved to Canada.

In 1979, while still in the U.K., I was elected Fellow of the Royal College of Surgeons of Edinburgh (FRCS Ed) and the Royal College of Physicians and Surgeons of Glasgow (FRCS Glas). As a surgeon I was called "Mister."

Unlike in North America, the surgeons in the U.K., Ireland and other Commonwealth countries are distinguished from physicians by being referred to as "Mister". The profession of surgery originated from barbers. Barber-surgeons were tradesmen. In the 18th century, barber-surgeons did not have any formal qualification unlike doctors who had university medical degrees.

This changed in the 19th century when the Royal College of Surgeons in London began to offer surgeons a formal status with college membership and fellowship. The title of "Mister" became a badge of honour for surgeons. A surgeon who has passed a fellowship examination of one of the Royal Colleges in the U.K. or Ireland is entitled to use the title of Mister, Miss, Mrs. or Ms.

I am also a Member of the Royal College of Physicians of London,

England and Licentiate of the Royal College of Surgeons of London, England (MRCP; LRCS).

I was single and life in England was good. Moving from hospital to hospital in strange cities was annoying and inconvenient but adventurous. Living in hospital residence was tolerable. Eating hospital food every day is not very appetizing. But years went by. I made lots of good friends and I am grateful to lots of people for looking after me and encouraging me to fulfill my dreams.

In Dartford, Barbara and Ken Groves and Sheila and John Lusher took good care of me. We are good friends and stay in touch.

I worked and trained under many surgeons in England who taught me what I know today. My chiefs at Hammersmith Hospital, Mr. John Castro and at Middlesborough General Hospital, Mr. Mike Cooke, became my good friends.

By the time I finished my training and got my surgical qualifications, I felt there was nothing more for me to do in England. Going back to Tanzania was not an option because of uncertainties created in East Africa by Uganda's brutal dictator, Idi Amin. My parents and the rest of the family had immigrated to U.K. and then to Canada.

After my surgical training I had one more learning desire. I wanted to get some experience in basic scientific research and publish some scientific papers. During one of my visits to Calgary, Canada, to see my parents, I met Dr. Martin Jerry, then Professor of Medicine at the University of Calgary and also Director of the Oncology Research Group at the Southern Alberta Cancer Clinic.

Jerry was looking for a Research Fellow and after an interview offered me a position. So I came to Canada on September 27, 1979 to work as a Research Fellow of the National Cancer Institute of Canada under the guidance of Dr. Martin Jerry at the Oncology Research Group. I was also a Scientific and Research Associate at the Southern Alberta Cancer Centre.

Those two years in Calgary were very enriching in many ways. I learned the Canadian way of life. Jerry was an outstanding mentor who guided me through some difficult times in establishing my credentials in Canada. I am ever so grateful to him and his lovely wife, Marian, for their kindness and generosity.

During my research years, I realized I could not practice as a specialist in general surgery in Canada without Canadian qualifications. After completing two years with Jerry, I was accepted as a surgical resident at the University of Alberta. Dr. Olin Thurston, then Director of the Surgical Residency Program, was very kind and helpful. The three years I spent in Edmonton were very difficult and frustrating. I had difficulty accepting the fact that all the years I spent in England, training to be a good surgeon, was not recognized here. People advised me to be patient. They said if I want to practice as a specialist in Canada I would have to obtain my Canadian qualifications. There is no short cut to it.

I saw these three years and more exams as a major roadblock to my eventual ambition of practicing as a surgeon. But I had no choice. I wanted to be recognized as a specialist, so I soldiered on. I had to be positive and look at those years as a stepping stone to my life in Canada.

With patience and perseverance I survived, thanks to many people in the residency program who were very kind and helpful. Some of them understood how I felt. Three years went by and I was elected fellow of the Royal College of Surgeons of Canada (FRCSC) in 1984 and Fellow of the American College of Surgeons (FACS) in 1989. I also became a Licentiate of the Medical Council of Canada (LMCC). I took numerous other exams to get to this point, but I was happy as this was the end of formal examinations for me.

So, after two years as a research fellow, two years as a surgical resident and one year as a surgical teaching fellow, and after having passed numerous Canadian examinations, I was now recognized as a qualified surgeon to practice in Canada. Wow! How many years of training, how many exams, how much sacrifice? Was it worth it?

Yes. It allowed me to be on equal footing with my colleagues who had Canadian surgical fellowship. I didn't have to spend the next 20 to 30 years thinking that I was not as good as my other surgical colleagues. What bothered me the most was the thought that before coming to Canada, I could perform surgery on people in the U.K. but was not considered good enough to operate in Canada as a specialist. I could have worked as a GP-surgeon in Saskatchewan and operated on Canadians living in Saskatchewan but not on Canadians living in Alberta or for that matter in British Columbia or some other provinces in Canada. Anyway, it is all behind me now. And I have been happy since receiving my Canadian surgical fellowship. I feel free.

During my research years in tumour immunology in Calgary, I developed an interest in the sub-specialty of surgical oncology. In 1983, during my year as a chief surgical resident, I had applied for a fellowship in surgical oncology at several U.S. programs. At that time there was only one program in Canada which was in its infancy, so Canada was not an option. I was delighted to be accepted at M.D. Anderson Hospital and Tumour Institute in Houston, Texas. After a couple of months I sent a message back to M.D. Anderson: "Houston, we have a problem!" Unfortunately I could not accept the position as I did not qualify for a U.S. visa to train at a U.S. hospital. So, that euphoria did not last too long. I must have been destined to work in North Battleford, Saskatchewan, and Medicine Hat, Alberta.

I was relatively old by the time I started my practice as a general surgeon in 1984. I was 39. After a year in North Battleford, I moved to Medicine Hat.

In 1984, North Battleford had a population of about 13,000. The hospital was small and the amount of surgical work I could do as a specialist was limited. Medicine Hat was looking for a general surgeon and after a couple of exploratory visits, I felt Medicine Hat was my kind of city. It was not as big as Calgary or Edmonton and not as small as North Battleford. It had a population of about 30,000.

By 2005, Medicine Hat had almost doubled in size. After 20 years in Medicine Hat, I am proud to say my memories of my first few days in Medicine Hat are as vivid as yesterday. They are good memories. People of Medicine Hat have been good to us and made us feel at home. And I am proud to be a Hatter!

I have a good surgical practice. I was Regional Chief of Medical Staff for the Palliser Health Region for close to four years. I enjoyed my work with the physicians and hospital administration. I am now semi-retired and do office consultations and procedures only.

Besides staying busy with my practice and family life, I have been involved in some community activities. Since 1985, I have been a volunteer and a fundraiser for the Medicine Hat branch of the Canadian Cancer Society. I have been the society's medical adviser, director, vice-president, president and provincial board member.

On May 30, 2003, I became the first physician in Medicine Hat to participate in Docs for Cancer by having my head shaved bald to raise funds for the Cancer Society (photos can be seen on my website: www.nbharwani.com). In 1997, at the age of 10, my son Hussein did the same thing–shaved his head bald for the Cancer Society as part of Cops for Cancer.

Writing has been my passion since I was in high school. I have been writing bits and pieces of things since my college days. I am a newspaper junkie and over the years I have written a few newspaper articles and letters to editors. My most consistent writing started in 1998 for the *Medicine Hat News* under then managing editor Gordon Wright.

I was introduced to Gord by one of his ace reporters, Ajay Bhardwaj. Ajay used to cover the local health authority for the *News* when I was Regional Chief of Medical Staff for the Palliser Health Region.

Since then I have written a regular health and wellness column titled What's Up Doc? for the *News*. Gord is a good teacher. Gord and his wife, Sheri, who was then assistant managing editor, encouraged me and guided me and gave me lots of ideas on how to write a good newspaper column. Without them this book would not have been possible.

In the last few years, I have worked with different editors at the *Medicine Hat News*, including Doug Hintz, Leah Prestayko and Alisha Sims. They have been very courteous, kind and helpful. I appreciate their help. It is always nice to work with a good editor who cares. I have been very lucky to have some nice people to work with and help me improve my writing skills.

Occasionally, my articles have appeared in the *Medical Post*. I have made several television info-mercials titled Medical Moments for CHAT TV, a Medicine Hat television station, as part of my ongoing interest to educate the public on health matters.

Medicine Hat has been a wonderful city for us. I enjoy my practice and raising children here has been fun. These days I indulge quite a bit in golfing, skiing, photography, travelling and, of course, writing. I would have never dreamt a little boy, who played on the shores of Lake Victoria, would one day call Medicine Hat, on the South Saskatchewan River, his home!

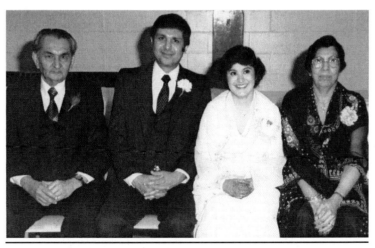

1983 – With my parents on my wedding day, April 1, 1983 (April Fool's Day).

Dr. Noorali Bharwani

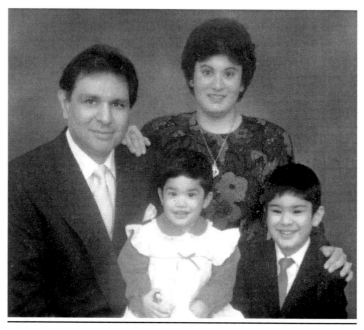

1991 – With my wife Sabiya and children: Alia 2 years old and Hussein 4 years old.

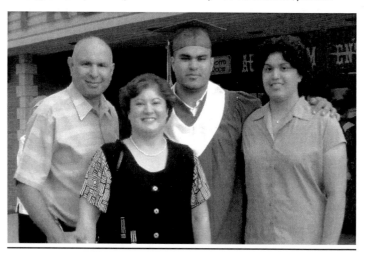

2005 – Hussein's high school graduation picture: Noorali, Sabiya, Hussein and Alia.

2

✳

Changing gears

From a surgeon to a physician-administrator

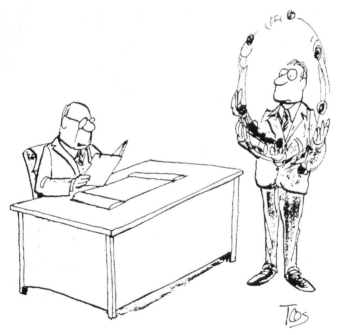

*"In addition to your juggling, what other background
do you have in medical management?"*

JULY-AUGUST 1998 **STITCHES**

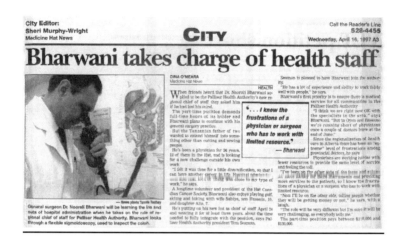

City Editor:
Sheri Murphy-Wright
Medicine Hat News

CITY

Call the Reader's Line
528-4455
Wednesday, April 16, 1997 A3

Bharwani takes charge of health staff

DINA O'MEARA
Medicine Hat News

When friends heard that Dr. Noorali Bharwani applied to be the Palliser Health Authority's new regional chief of staff they asked him if he had lost his mind.

The part-time position demands full-time hours of its holder and Bharwani plans to continue with his general surgery practice.

But the Tanzanian father of two wanted to extend himself into something other than cutting and sewing people.

He's been a physician for 26 years, 13 of them in the Hat, and is looking for a new challenge outside his own work.

"I felt it was time for a little diversification, so that I can have another career in life. Hospital administration also fits into my type of work," he says.

A longtime volunteer and president of the Hat Canadian Cancer Society Bharwani also enjoys playing golf, skiing and hiking with wife Sabiya, son Hussein, 18, and daughter Alia, 7.

He's putting on his new hat as chief of staff April 24 and weaning it for at least three years, about the time needed to fully integrate with the position, says Palliser Health Authority president Tom Seaman.

HEALTH

"*. . . I know the frustrations of a physician or surgeon who has to work with limited resource.*"
— Bharwani

Seaman is pleased to have Bharwani join the authority.

"He has a lot of experience and ability to work fairly well with people," he says.

Bharwani's first priority is to ensure there is medical service for all communities in the Palliser Health Authority

"I think we are right near OK with the specialists in the area," says Bharwani. "But in Oyen and Bassano we're running short of physicians once a couple of doctors leave at the end of June."

Since the regionalization of health care in Alberta there has been an "extreme" level of frustrations among provincial doctors, he says.

Physicians are working harder with fewer resources to provide the same level of service and feeling the toll.

"I've been on the other side of the fence and I know the frustrations of a physician or surgeon who has to work with limited resource.

"Now I'll be on the other side, telling people whether they will be getting money or not," he says, with a laugh.

"The role will be very different but I'm sure it will be very challenging, as everybody tells me."

The part-time position pays between $110,000 and $130,000.

— News photo Tannis Toohey

General surgeon Dr. Noorali Bharwani will be learning the ins and outs of hospital administration when he takes on the role of regional chief of staff for Palliser Health Authority. Bharwani looks through a flexible sigmoidoscopy, used to inspect the colon.

In 1996, at the age of 51, I had my first episode of angina. It happened on a Thursday, which used to be my operating room (OR) day. I was doing a major abdominal surgery on a young patient with Peutz-Jeghers Syndrome (PJS). PJS is a rare disorder of the gastro-intestinal tract that is inherited from a parent or occurs spontaneously. Patients with PJS develop complications from intestinal and gastric polyps.

It was a busy week. I was in OR almost every day performing major bowel surgeries. On that particular Thursday, I was on my last case when I developed severe upper back pain. I began sweating. Upper back pain is not unusual for me. I am tall and I have a hump. But this was different.

I called on one of my general surgical colleagues to come and finish my case for me. My surgical assistant was Dr. Noel Hassett. He was also my family physician at that time. He asked me to go to emergency room and have a cardiogram done. After the blood tests and cardiogram, the ER physician and the internist on call felt I should be admitted to the intensive care unit for observation. They suspected the pain in the upper back was due to my coronaries.

Within a few days I was flown to Calgary. I had an angiogram, which confirmed the presence of coronary artery disease. I had immediate angioplasty.

This was a wake-up call, a lucky one too! I could have dropped dead in the operating room. A voice in my head said, "Doctor, heal thyself."

On my way back to Medicine Hat and for a few days after, I spent some time reflecting on my future. I had a wife and two young children. I wanted to see my children grow and hopefully obtain a university education. I was hoping to be there to help them achieve their ambitions. I felt it was time to slow down and take care of myself and my family.

But there is no easy way out for a sick doctor who wants to slow down, especially for a surgeon whose main job satisfaction and income comes from performing major surgeries and making sick patients feel better. As one of my colleagues told me, once a surgeon, always a surgeon, and he knew how much I loved doing surgery. He believed that I would not be happy doing anything else. But the stress of after-hour demands related to on-call schedules was tough on me.

I wasn't getting enough sleep. I was scared to die suddenly from a heart attack. But there was no room for a part-time surgeon, either you provide a full-meal deal or quit. So I explored other ideas.

I felt to stay healthy I should do something of interest to me, keep me reasonably busy, and provide me with a reasonable income and a reasonable lifestyle.

At this time the job of Regional Chief of Medical Staff (RCOS) for the Palliser Health Authority became vacant. This is an administrative position. It is a combination of being a physician manager and a liaison officer between the health authority and the physicians, a sort of messenger and enforcer of medical staff by-laws who gets shot from both sides if things don't go right! This was advertised as a half-time administrative position. I applied, and I was hired.

Some people thought I was crazy to apply for the job. They said it would be more stressful than working round the clock as a surgeon and it would not be good for my health.

I wasn't worried about that at all. I knew it was a challenging and interesting job. I knew the people I would be working with in the administration were nice and friendly. I knew there would be a certain amount of time needed to understand the issues involved. I knew it was a sensitive position in terms of medical staff politics and issues involved in dealing with your own colleagues. However, I had full faith in my physician colleagues. I knew they would respect me if I was open and fair with them.

I started my work as RCOS in April 1997. I gradually quit my hospital work and maintained some out-patient office practice. I thought I would never go back to active surgical practice. Although the RCOS job was advertised as a part-time job, I soon realized it was more than that. I devoted all my energies to make this a successful endeavour. I wanted to make some changes and I knew there were many challenges.

Years went by pretty fast. I was there for close to four years (three years and eight months to be precise).

It was hard work. There were tough times and disappointments. I had to be patient and diplomatic but overall it was a satisfactory endeavour.

My boss and CEO of Palliser Health Authority, Tom Seaman, was a thorough gentleman with an excellent sense of humour and skills in quiet diplomacy. The chairman of the regional board, John Boksteyn, was a good, forward-looking man, dedicated to his work. I received wonderful support from the members of the health board, the administration and the hospital staff in Medicine Hat and from the rest of the region.

In Marg Degen, I had a very experienced executive assistant. The vast majority of the physicians were very helpful, understanding and co-operative. It is impossible to be a successful physician manager without getting help from all the parties you are trying to help. I was lucky in the amount of goodwill I received from various quarters.

We had good success in recruiting doctors and creating an environment where doctors could work amicably especially in small places such as Oyen, Brooks, Bassano and Bow Island. We recruited enough specialists and family physicians, to complement what we already had, to work in Medicine Hat, a regional referral centre.

We were able to put in place new medical staff bylaws and rules and reorganized committee structures. This is a very important requirement for risk management and patient safety.

We were able to increase interaction and communication between the physicians, hospital administration and the regional board by organizing social functions and meetings outside the hospital setting.

A monthly newsletter (*The Way I See It—from the Regional Chief of Staff*) was created to inform the physicians about the happenings in the region and the province. Budget information was shared with the physicians and their input was solicited. The newsletter offered information, jokes, cartoons and some words of wisdom.

We were able to make many other positive changes which are difficult to list here as they would be of minimal interest to non-physicians.

Years were going by rapidly. I had given a commitment to work for three years. I was into my fourth year and I felt it was time to move on and allow somebody else to bring in new ideas and new energy. After much hesitation I gave my resignation in December 2000. I returned to my surgical practice.

I was sad to say goodbye to my colleagues in the administration. I enjoyed working with them and with my physician colleagues. They are all hardworking dedicated people trying to achieve the same results: good patient care and safety. I wish them well.

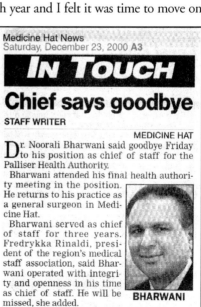

Medicine Hat News
Saturday, December 23, 2000 **A3**

IN TOUCH

Chief says goodbye

STAFF WRITER

MEDICINE HAT

Dr. Noorali Bharwani said goodbye Friday to his position as chief of staff for the Palliser Health Authority.

Bharwani attended his final health authority meeting in the position. He returns to his practice as a general surgeon in Medicine Hat.

Bharwani served as chief of staff for three years. Fredrykka Rinaldi, president of the region's medical staff association, said Bharwani operated with integrity and openness in his time as chief of staff. He will be **BHARWANI** missed, she added.

The search for a replacement for Bharwani is continuing, PHA president Tom Seaman said Friday.

3

※

Dead man walking

Ten years after changing gears

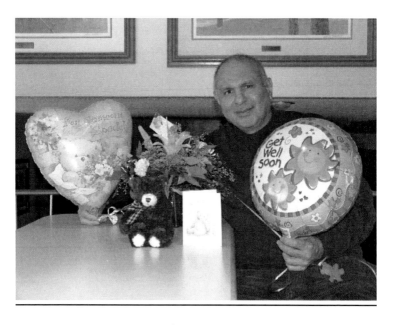

January, 2006
Noorali recuperating at home after hospitalization in Medicine Hat and Calgary

Life is what happens to us while we are making other plans.

~ Thomas La Mance

On Wednesday, January 17, 2006 I was sitting in the intensive care unit (ICU) of the Medicine Hat Regional Hospital (MHRH) feeling sorry for myself. I wasn't there as a doctor but as a patient. An impatient patient.

This is what happened. The previous day, Tuesday, I was driving to work and had severe chest pain. I felt unwell. I reached my office and felt my condition getting worse. So I turned back and went straight to the hospital emergency department. I was stabilized and then admitted to ICU.

You see, I had been under the weather for the previous couple of weeks. But like a typical male-patient and a doctor-patient, I was taking my time to visit my family physician. I thought it was a recurrence of angina and I started using nitroglycerine spray to relieve the symptoms. There did not appear to be any urgency to rush to ER although my wife felt that I should be in the hospital. I was planning to see my family doctor and my cardiologist in the near future as my symptoms did not feel that bad. As you may recall from the previous chapter, my last episode of angina was about 10 years ago. Since then I have had cardiac rhythm problems but no angina.

Recently, my health appeared to be in excellent condition. I felt 2005 was a good year for me in many ways. I was lucky to have many wonderful things happen to me. I always try to adhere to the principles of ELMOSS (exercise, laughter, meditation, organic healthy food, stress relief and no smoking). And my plan was to continue to adhere to these principles for 2006.

But somebody had different plans for me. As I drove to work that day, I realized I needed help. I could not postpone it anymore. The chest pain wasn't going away with nitroglycerine and the pain was recurring every few minutes. My right shoulder and right arm felt very uncomfortable and my back needed stretching all the time. I could not get comfortable. Patients with classical symptoms of heart attack and angina have pain radiating to the left shoulder and arm. Mine was on the right side.

So here I was, lying on an ICU bed with oxygen prongs in my nostrils. Millions of cables from my hairy chest (ouch) were connected to the cardiac monitor. An intravenous catheter was in my right wrist, a name tag and allergy tag on my left wrist.

My vital signs were monitored every two hours. Blood tests were ordered at frequent intervals to check if I had a heart attack. Thank goodness they don't use rectal thermometers anymore. And not every patient admitted to the hospital needs an enema these days. At least we have made some scientific progress in that direction.

My smiling nurses and physicians kept me stable and amused with their care and visits. My wife and children were concerned but very supportive and patient. Their visits and visits from my friends were a great strength to me.

But I still felt miserable and sorry for myself. The invincible Dr. B was in hospital again. I had to cancel my office duties and several procedures for the rest of the week. Some patients had gone through that ghastly bowel prep for their colon check in my office that day. They will have to drink the stuff again.

I had to cancel several vasectomies for that week. These young fellows take time off and get themselves psyched up for the procedure. Now they will have to go through all that again. Several patients were to see me for consultations and follow-up. They will have to wait little longer. For the last couple of years I have maintained a low key office surgical practice so I did not have to cancel any major surgical procedures in the hospital.

"Doctor, heal thyself first," said my doctor. If I didn't get better now then I may not see any patients ever. I was diagnosed with unstable angina and I was lucky to be alive. I tried to be a model patient and the plan was to transfer me to Calgary for an urgent angiogram. Next day, on Thursday, a bed was found for me and I was flown by air ambulance to Foothills Hospital (FHH) in Calgary.

Angina is a condition in which chest pain occurs with exertion because coronary vessels are narrow and the blood supply (carrying oxygen and nutrients) to the heart muscle is compromised. I was diagnosed with unstable angina. Unstable angina is a condition in which chest pain occurs at rest or with minimal activity but the heart muscle is not damaged as it would have been if I had a heart attack. Within an hour or two of arriving at FHH, I underwent coronary angiography. This is an imaging technique in which X-ray pictures are taken to visualize the inner opening of blood filled structures, including arteries, veins and the heart chambers. My angiogram showed two areas of narrowing in the right coronary artery. Immediate angioplasties and insertion of two stents were carried out to keep the blood flow to the heart.

Angioplasty is carried out by inserting a balloon-tipped catheter (thin tube) in the diseased narrowed blood vessel. The balloon stretches the blood vessel improving blood flow through it. A stent is a mesh of thin metal which helps keep the blood vessel open.

That night I was kept on Unit 103B of the FHH for close observation to monitor for any complications like chest pain or bleeding from the groin where the catheter was inserted. My stay was uneventful. Next day I was transferred to Unit 4W substation at the MHRH for more observation and blood tests. I was discharged the following day which was a Saturday.

I was lucky that I did not have a heart attack or a stroke. I was fortunate to have everything done in five days. I was very happy with the attention and care I received in Medicine Hat and Calgary.

What do I have to worry about now?

It is important to remember that coronary angioplasty and insertion of a stent is not a cure for coronary artery disease (CAD). Research shows that narrowing in the coronary artery will recur within six months in one out of five people who have had coronary angioplasty. My aim will be to prevent this from happening.

How can I do that?

I should try and control the process called atherosclerosis. Athero in

Greek means paste and sclerosis means hardening. In atherosclerosis, there is a deposit of fatty substances, cholesterol and other substances to form a plaque which makes the blood vessel narrow. Atherosclerosis is usually a slow, complex disease that typically starts in childhood and often progresses when people grow older. Like arthritis, it is a progressive disease.

The underlying risk factors for atherosclerosis are:

- family history of heart disease
- high bad cholesterol (LDL)
- exposure to tobacco smoke
- high blood pressure
- diabetes mellitus
- obesity and
- physical inactivity.

The only risk factor I have is bad genes. I cannot change that. My LDL is within normal range but my cardiologist wants me to reduce it further. This can only be done with pills. I am not obese but I can afford to lose some weight. Otherwise, I don't have other risk factors.

It is hard to predict the future. The recovery process was slow. I felt physically and emotionally wounded. I thought I was doing everything right but looks like it wasn't good enough. I had started 2006 with confidence and big plans for the year to ski, golf, take holidays and continue with my office practice. But the attack of angina was a rude awakening and a reminder that you cannot take life for granted and one should never lower his or her guard in good times or bad times.

I am now on more medications than before. I will have to watch my bad cholesterol on a more frequent basis. I will have to exercise more. I will lose some more weight although I am not overweight. I will be more careful what I eat. I will further reduce stress in my life. Who knows I may live a long life.

Wellness is the key to a long and healthy life.
Many people have the wrong perception of it.
Wellness is from the neck up, and fitness from the neck down.
Too many people work out every day, but go around with the worst
attitudes, which just wastes all their physical efforts.
~ Golf Quote from my friend Tony

4

What's Up Doc?

Writing for the Medicine Hat News

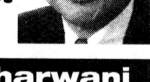

My purpose in writing a column......is to stimulate people to think about what I consider fairly important issues. It does not matter to me if people agree or disagree. I don't pretend to be omniscient, and, in fact, I am no smarter than anybody else.
~ Charley Reese, Orlando Sentinel, December 27th, 1998

It was the summer of 1998 when I had a meeting with Gordon Wright, then managing editor of the *Medicine Hat News*. With his help and encouragement, my first column, *"What's Up Doc?"* appeared in the News on August 13, 1998.

It is hard to believe so many years have gone by. But I enjoy writing. Since 1998, I have written many columns. I have occasionally written for the *Medical Post* as well. My columns also appear in *Oyen Echo*.

I wrote my first newspaper article when I was a medical student in Patna, India. The newspaper was called *Searchlight*. The article was published on November 19, 1967. Since then I have written numerous letters to editors and have published articles on a random basis in different newspapers. I am a newspaper junkie and follow politics nationally and internationally quite closely.

My most consistent writing has been for the *Medicine Hat News*. The purpose of writing the column is to help the reader understand the various aspects of health care spiced with a local touch and some humour.

I look at the medical journals and listen to people's health concerns and discuss what is new and what is important.

I try to explain to readers why it is important to take certain proactive preventive measures to live a happy, stress free and healthy life.

I try to explain medicine is not a perfect science and doctors are like any human beings – from time to time vulnerable to making mistakes.

My columns have been sometimes serious, sometimes lighthearted but hopefully simple, educational and current. I hope they have not been outrageous or divisive. I apply the principles of 4Cs – the column has to be clear, concise, correct and complete.

Writing the column has also been a selfish endeavor. Teaching is the best way to learn. Sharing knowledge is the best way to improve one's self. In the process I have learned a lot about myself, my health and my own deficiencies.

I have tried to follow what I write and in the process I have made significant changes in my own lifestyle. One change at a time has added up to a better and more satisfactory lifestyle. Rome wasn't built in a day. So there is still hope to achieve nirvana, an ideal condition of rest, harmony, stability and joy.

The column which generated the most response and comments from the readers was the one about my mother – her brief life history and battle with a large benign brain tumour. Old age can be cruel and right now she is praying very hard for nirvana.

ELMOSS (exercise, laughter, meditation, organic healthy foods, stress relief, and do not smoke) has been my guiding principle. I have written many columns on this subject.

Many other subjects have been covered in these columns. Space does not allow me to mention them all. But I have posted them all on my website (www.nbharwani.com).

Writing is a dangerous and contagious disease and I am infected with it! But the point of good writing is knowing when to stop (L.M.Montgomery). So, let me end this chapter by saying thank you to the *Medicine Hat News* and to the readers for their support.

It is in the hard rockpile labour of seeking to win, hold, or deserve a reader's interest that the pleasant agony of writing comes in.
~ John Mason Brown

Plaudits to Dr. Bharwani

I am always looking forward to "What's up doc?" — Dr. Bharwani's column on health. It offers such good advice and is easily understood.

He has great concern about the well-being of people. Thank you Dr. Bharwani.

Doris Hoogestraat
Medicine Hat

Letter to editor, the Medicine Hat News, August 18, 1999

Letter to editor, the *Medicine Hat News*, August 18, 1999

5

A tower of strength

The world always needs fathers who give guidance
by the lives they live.
~ Unknown Author

I wrote this article for Father's Day, 2002. This was and is a tribute not only to my father but all the fathers who make so many sacrifices to raise their children. No parent is perfect. We all make mistakes, but in the end what separates a good person is the recognition that he or she cares.

Here is what I had to say:

Father's day is a day to appreciate our fathers. A father is appreciated for many things. For his sacrifices. For teaching his children the right stuff. For preparing them to survive the constant danger they face. And for being there when he is needed.

With close to a 50 per cent divorce rate in developed countries, through illness and accident, many children have been deprived of their fathers. For them this day becomes even more special – to ask why life is unfair and what we can do to make this world a better place to live.

My father, Hussein, died on February 4, 1991 in Calgary. He was 79 years old. He died the way he wanted to go – suddenly. He had a heart attack.

Hussein had his fair share of ups and downs in his life. Let me share with you Hussein's journey through four continents in search of safety, security, prosperity and happiness for his family.

Hussein was born in Gujarat, India. He joined the work force at the early age of 13, when, in 1924, he came to Tanzania (then Tanganyika) from India with his older brother. His father's business in India had failed, the local economy was bad, and the family needed financial help. So Hussein, after finishing Grade 4, embarked on a voyage of adventure to find work in Africa.

It took him almost a month by boat across the Indian Ocean and by rail across East Africa to arrive in Bukoba, on the shores of Lake Victoria, Tanzania. For eight years, Hussein and his brother ran a clothing store in Bukoba and sent money to their father so he could support the rest of the family.

At the age of 21, Hussein went back to India to look for a bride. He married Sikina. Hussein stayed two years in Gujarat and their first child, Gulshan, was born. Sikina stayed to look after Gulshan and the in-laws, and Hussein went back to Tanzania. This time he went to Musoma, another small town on the shores of Lake Victoria. He found a job, and Sikina and Gulshan joined him two years later when Hussein had saved enough money to bring them over.

Hussein was becoming restless again and wanted to start his own business. He did this in Kinesi, a small town across the river from Musoma. After five years in Kinesi, Hussein moved back to Musoma to continue expanding his business. Hussein's family was growing in number (four girls and four boys). With the family manpower he had, at one time Hussein was running three shops in a fairly small town.

Life as a businessman was not always rosy. There were ups and downs. After 25 years in Musoma, he made another move to a bigger town, Mwanza on Lake Victoria. Mwanza had a high school and it was good for his children. Perhaps Hussein's best legacy was to encourage and support his children to seek more knowledge and strive for university education. For a man who had only a Grade 4

education, Hussein knew the value of higher learning: security.
Then came the era of Idi Amin and his terror in Uganda. In 1972,
after 15 years in Mwanza, Hussein had to move again, first to England
(three years) and then to Canada. Hussein and Sikina settled in
Calgary.

As Hussein got older, he suffered from several health problems.
He had heart disease for 20 years and was in pain with rheumatoid
arthritis. But he was a very strong, handsome, tall man. His appearance
defied his internal sufferings.

He feared no one but God and lived a very clean, sensible life. He
believed in caring, loving and giving. He was a tower of strength to his
family. He had no unfinished business left when he was summoned
to his last journey on February 4, 1991. He knew he had fulfilled all
his obligations as a father. At the end he was a satisfied man, at peace
with himself. A job well done!

May his soul rest in eternal peace. Amen.

Hussein Jina Bharwani (1911-1991)

6

Isn't she lovely!

What the mother sings to the cradle
goes all the way down to the coffin.
~ Henry Ward Beecher (1813-1887)

In May 2000, in one of my newspaper columns, I wrote about a very special lady. A lady, who has been a very important part of my life. A lady, who has taught me many things.

Here is what I had to say about her life:

Allow me to tell you a story of a very special, tough and courageous 84-year-old lady. Her name is Sikina. In the year 2000, she spent five weeks in Foothills Hospital in Calgary for removal of a six centimeter benign brain tumour. The tumour had left her partially paralyzed.

Sikina was born in India. At the very tender age of 15 she married a young handsome fellow named Hussein, who was 21. At the age of 13, Hussein had gone to East Africa with his older brother to look for work. After eight years of work and making some money, he had returned to India to look for a bride. That is when he was introduced to Sikina and got married.

Hussein and Sikina lived in East Africa for many years. They had eight children. One day, in 1965, Sikina was travelling from Tanzania to Uganda (to attend to her daughter Gulshan's delivery) when her car was involved in a head-on collision with a drunk driver. She sustained life-threatening injuries to her head, face, right thigh and both arms. Many of her bones were broken.

Sikina never gave up. With Hussein at her bedside, she fought back and survived. She spent four months in a hospital in Kampala, Uganda. She came home to Tanzania walking with crutches. After another two months of physiotherapy she was back taking care of her family.

With Idi Amin's brutal regime in Uganda, the political atmosphere in East Africa became very uncertain. So, in 1975, Hussein, Sikina and their children moved to Calgary.

Five years later, Sikina developed right-sided weakness. She was found to have a brain tumour close to a large blood vessel. Two neurosurgeons in Calgary felt nothing should be done, as there was a significant risk of damaging the blood vessel during surgery which could be fatal.

Hussein wasn't a man to give up easily. As Sikina's condition worsened, Hussein insisted on another opinion. The third neurosurgeon, after considerable deliberation and consultation with his colleagues at the Calgary General Hospital, elected to do the surgery. This was in 1980. Sikina and her family were warned of the likely complications. But Sikina was ready for it, as she could not live the way she felt.

Sikina survived the six-hour surgery. She had a full recovery. Eighty per cent of the tumour was removed. Luckily it was benign. The portion of the tumour close to the blood vessel was left behind.

After many years of good health, Sikina's troubles started again. Her right leg was getting weaker. Then in April 2000, she momentarily lost her speech and function on the right side of her body. She was thought to have had a stroke and rushed to Foothills Hospital in Calgary. Investigations revealed the recurrence of a large tumour at the site of the previous excision.

Within a week, she was back in the operating room undergoing another six hours of brain surgery. This time the recovery was slow. She was in the hospital for five weeks. But she did not give up!

Now she is home looking better and walking with a walker. Another courageous fight and a miraculous recovery! This time Hussein wasn't there. He passed away in 1991. But all her children and their families were there. So were the neurosurgeons, anesthetist, geriatrician, nursing staff and physiotherapists. It was excellent teamwork.

Sikina believes in God and miracles. But one thing stands out—Sikina's courage. I am proud of her. She is a special lady. And she is my mother!

Sikina Hussein Bharwani (born 1920)

7

Walking and my grandma

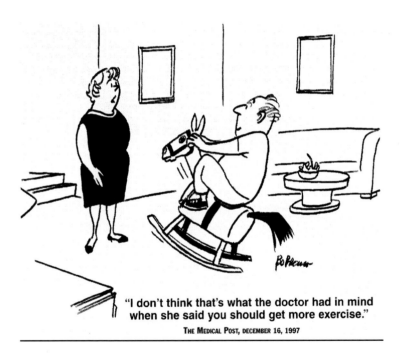

"I don't think that's what the doctor had in mind
when she said you should get more exercise."

THE MEDICAL POST, DECEMBER 16, 1997

After dinner, rest a while. After supper, walk a mile.

~ an Arab saying

Walking is wonderful exercise. My grandmother started walking 10 kilometres a day when she was 60. Now she is 100 years old and we don't know where the hell she is!

Ok, don't worry, that is not true. We know where she is. She is somewhere in heaven, probably looking down and smiling at me and at my silly little joke. The joke is from one of many e-mails I receive where some jokes are really funny and some are really stupid. I guess stupidity is meant to be funny.

Come to think of it, my grandma did like walking. Quite often there was no choice. We lived in the small towns of Musoma and Mwanza on the shores of Lake Victoria in Tanzania. The best mode of transportation was our legs or bikes. We did not own a car. We walked or biked everywhere.

As a young boy, I remember holding my grandma's hand helping her walk through the dark alleys and the roads of those small towns. There was no electricity. We used a flash light or kerosene lanterns.

Every evening my grandma would go to a prayer hall to pray and meditate. In fact, we would all go as a family every single day. One of us was put in charge of her safety. Those were the days of large extended families where we all looked after each other. There was nothing like nursing homes, group homes or assisted living. We took care of our own.

My grandma was 81 years old when she died. She had a severe case of asthma.

Medicine Hat reminds me of Musoma and Mwanza except it is bigger. It is small enough to have everything within walking distance but how many of us walk to work or to go shopping?

Of course there are exceptions. Everybody is not lazy like me. There are lots of people who walk or bike to work and go shopping. And there are many people for whom using a vehicle is important for health and safety reasons.

Walking is not always easy. Changing weather and flu season is a hindrance to establish consistent walking habit. We are so seasonal in everything we do in a year that our brains are frozen in that mentality.

And icy roads and sidewalks are dangerous.

But we do have many good days in Medicine Hat. The majority of the people (including me) should be able to walk to most of the places. But the problem is we are always in a hurry to get to our destination and then rush back home. We never seem to stop and ask, "Why am I rushing? Why cannot I take my time and enjoy the walk?"

So, slow down and start walking. You can walk leisurely 30 minutes a day for general health benefits. You can walk briskly to improve cardiovascular fitness by walking 30 minutes a day five days a week. If you are trying to lose weight then you need to walk briskly for 45 to 60 minutes a day five days a week. And make sure your dinners are slimmer.

Be like my grandma......... walk, walk, walk and be healthy and happy. You may even go to heaven!

Walking is the best possible exercise.
Habituate yourself to walk very far.
~ Thomas Jefferson 1743-1826

Shambai Jina Punja Bharwani, born in 1891 in Kalanda Gondal in Gujarat, India and died in 1972 in Tanzania at the age of 81.

8

Cancer kills a Canadian dream

The dream, alone, is of interest. What is life, without a dream?
~ Edmond Rostand (1868-1918)

My sister Gulshan was 10 years older than me. She was the first of the eight children my parents had. She was born on June 25, 1935 in Jamjodhpur, Gujarat, India. At that time my mother was only 16 years old. My mother moved to Tanzania to join my dad when Gulshan was two years old.

As years went by, Gulshan gradually took over the responsibility of looking after her younger brothers and sisters as my parents got more busy running businesses in Musoma. She did an excellent job of looking after us before she married and had a large family of her own. We have many fond memories of her. She was a great help to my mom and dad. She was like a second mother to the rest of the siblings.

Gulshan was very kind, caring and religious. She was very hard working. She was an excellent cook.

On September 14, 1996 she died of pancreatic cancer within three months of diagnosis. We have no family history of any kind of cancer. We have a family history of heart disease and Gulshan had chronic atrial fibrillation (irregular heart beat). Her cardiac condition had nothing to do with her death.

She suffered from abdominal discomfort for some time. Every time she saw her doctor or went to the emergency department, the doctors would worry more about her heart than the abdomen. So when she was finally diagnosed with pancreatic cancer, it came as shock to the rest of the family. They were told the prognosis was bad.

The family felt something more should be done to save her. She was under the care of one of the top surgeons in the country who specialized in pancreatic and biliary surgery. Gulshan was booked for surgery several times but it was always cancelled because the operating rooms were always fully booked. By the time she had surgery she was full of cancer and nothing more could be done.

Pancreatic cancer is the fifth leading cause of cancer death in North America. The prognosis is dismal. The overall five-year survival rate is less than two per cent, the worst of any cancer. Only 20 per cent of patients will be diagnosed at a stage where surgery may offer hope.

The surgery is extensive, with significant complications. Even for those who survive the ordeal, the five-year prognosis may not be better than 25 per cent.

Why is it difficult to make an early diagnosis?

Two main reasons: first, the pancreas is a long, narrow, transverse, deep-seated organ behind the stomach in the upper abdomen; second, the initial symptoms are none or very vague. By the time ultrasound or CAT scan picks it up, it is too late.

What causes pancreatic cancer?

The precise cause is unknown. Smoking and chronic inflammation are suspected in the causation of the disease. An estimated 5-10 per cent of pancreatic cancers are inherited and an additional 10-20 per cent may have other significant genetic influence.

Over the previous 25 years, Gulshan and her husband, Madat, had overcome many difficulties. They had to run away from Idi Amin's brutality and arrived penniless as refugees from Uganda with six children. The youngest, triplets, were about a year old.

They were in Quebec for a couple of years and then moved to Vancouver. Madat is a good watch repairer. After moving from a few unsatisfactory jobs, he opened his own business, a jewelry shop. Gulshan ran the shop and Madat repaired watches. They were happy. They were looking forward to retirement and travelling as their children were growing and leaving home one at a time. They also enjoyed their grandchildren.

As parents, they had their share of problems raising children. Their oldest daughter, Rozmin developed multiple sclerosis soon after she had two children of her own. Now Rozmin is totally disabled. That is another tragedy the family has to deal with.

Now Gulshan is gone and so are her dreams. She wanted to go back and visit Quebec to thank all the people who had helped her settle in Canada. She could not do it. She wanted to visit the U.K. as she had never been there. She could not do it. She wanted to help look after Rozmin's children and her interests. She could not do it.

Sixty is a young age to die. But who knows how and when cancer is going to strike you. All we can do is have dreams, live a reasonably healthy life, work hard and hope for the best. We should not postpone to tomorrow what we can do today. Life can be short. And dreams can be even shorter. But dreams are always interesting. That is why we all have dreams.

Did anyone ever have a boring dream?
~ Ralph Hodgson (1871-1962)

Gulshan Dharamshi (1935-1996)

9

Oh, God! What's your game plan?

And almost everyone when age, disease or sorrows strike him, inclines to
think there is a God, or something very like Him.
~ Arthur Hugh Clough (1819-1861)

In many respects, year 2001 was not a good one. In fact, it is difficult
to look back at 2001 and say anything nice.

Once upon a time we thought that the world was shrinking. "It's a
small world," was one of the most commonly used phrases. I haven't
heard this sentence recently. Now even the U.S. feels distant! Travel
across the border is not taken for granted.

Worldwide, there is news of death and destruction, of fear, terror
and revenge.

Human differences have never been verbalized or written about so
much. Are my fears different than yours? Is my God different than
my neighbour's? Are these differences important when millions of
people are dying from illness, wars, starvation and terrorism? Is their
God different than yours or mine?

Closer to home, many families lost their loved ones due to sickness
or accident. In Medicine Hat, medical and nursing staff of Palliser
Health Region lost three of their finest: Dr. Ivan Witt, Dr. Keith
Clugston and Nurse Wendy Smith. It was a big loss not only to their
families but also to their colleagues and patients. What is more painful

they were taken away from us so suddenly. They were relatively young and were providing much needed service in the community and to their families. What did their God have in mind?

Then there are people in hospitals or at home who are chronically ill and incapacitated. They are waiting to die because they are in pain. They are suffering. One such person was my 88-year-old mother-in-law who lived in Vancouver. For several weeks she had been close to death. She continued to live but her end was so near but so far. The family waited and flew in and out of Vancouver not knowing what to do.

If there was a case for euthanasia, here was one. Her body was small and frail. All the body fat had disappeared. The joints were stiff and painful. The bedsores were bad and hard to watch. The muscles were wasting away. She was unable to eat or drink. She was literally starving to death.

Morphine helped relieve her pain. Her dutiful son, John, who had looked after her for so many years, waited and watched in helpless despair. "What can I do to make it easy for my mother without prolonging her sufferings?" he kept on asking. The best thing was to keep her pain free and comfortable. But it was painful to watch. He maintained a round-the-clock vigil. He wanted to be at the bedside until the end. She died soon after Christmas that year.

My father-in-law died from prostate cancer and old age some years ago. He suffered for many years as well. His old age was not very good. Again John sacrificed a lot to look after him. I knew my in-laws when I was in boarding school in Dar-es-Salaam. They looked after me well. They were very religious and devoted many years to community service. They were generous and helped many people. I thought they deserved a better, healthier and pain free old age. But they did not get one. I wonder why. Why did God not have a better plan for them?

We know life isn't fair. Whether it is your God or mine, He has His game plan. There isn't much we can do except learn to be decent human beings by sharing and enjoying what we have with those who are struggling in life. I think the God of the Christians, Jews, Muslims, Hindus, Buddhists, and others teach the same thing—be nice and help others.

Time and again we have learned that life is too short. But greed and exploitation continues. Yesterday's friends are enemies today. And yesterday's enemies are friends today. It is no secret that ruthless exploiters (I wonder if their God is different than yours or mine) take full advantage of the majority of the people who are honest, decent and God-fearing individuals.

Trying to understand God is not easy. There are so many questions but no reasonable answers. It's all about faith. And a God-fearing religious person like me is not supposed to question God and His motives. So, let's get on with life!

> *What men usually ask of God when they pray*
> *is that two and two not make four.*
> ~ Anonymous

Hassanali Kassum Sunderji (1912-1999)
Nurbanu Hassanali Kassum Sunderji (1913-2001)

10

Gifts of love and caring

The individual succumbs, but he does not die
if he has left something to mankind.
~ Will Durant (1885-198)

On August 18, 2001, I was one of the hundreds of people who packed the Medicine Hat College Theatre to bid final goodbye to my friend and partner, Dr. Ivan Witt.

Ivan was larger than life. He worked hard and thoroughly enjoyed the fruits of his labour. He cared about his family, friends and patients. Many of us will miss his sense of humour, and zest for life and work. Ivan's sudden and premature death affected people in many different ways.

It was in the afternoon of Sunday August 4, 2001, when my phone rang. I could not believe what I heard – that Ivan and his family were involved in a motor vehicle collision and Ivan had died at the scene. My mind immediately flashed back to Sunday, October 14, 1984, when my phone rang at about 10 p.m. to let me know my younger brother, Mansur, was killed in a motor vehicle collision near his home in Royston, B.C. At that time I was in North Battleford, Saskatchewan.

Mansur was 36. He had two young children: a girl, 7, and boy, 5. A few months prior to Mansur's death, his daughter Rehana had spent about six months in a Vancouver hospital with debilitating effects of viral infection of the brain. Mansur was a hard working young man devoted to his faith and his family. Now Mansur was gone. The family had to go through two major setbacks in one year. How many of us can understand the magnitude of the situation?

In another chapter I have already talked about my sister Gulshan. She came penniless to Canada as a refugee with six children (including one-year-old triplets) and started life in Quebec and then moved to Vancouver. Now her daughter is disabled with multiple sclerosis and Gulshan died from pancreatic cancer at the age of 60, many of her dreams still unfulfilled.

Unfortunately, almost every family has sad stories like these. But do we learn anything from these stories or by attending funeral services?

Certainly the message is quite clear. Life is too short and we are all going to die one day. If that is the case then why are we in this world? What is the purpose of our existence?

The answer to these questions comes in a tragic story I read in *Golf Digest*. This is the story of 45-year-old Pete Farricker, *Golf Digest*'s equipment editor. Pete was diagnosed with Lou Gehrig's disease. The author of the article says "the disease goes on to ravage the victim, in a cruel twist, shutting down the body while leaving the mind intact." While Pete was waiting to die, he wrote his own eulogy that was read by his wife at his funeral service.

In part this is what he said:

"...it was the never-ending gifts of love that came my way, which convinced me that the main reason why we're all here is to simply love one another. We all have what seem like complicated lives, and we often get caught up in the daily minutiae of work, family and school...it's love that makes us strong—and love that solves the mysteries."

Ivan, Mansur, and Gulshan were good examples of this. They loved their work. They loved their families. They loved the people they came in touch with. But now they are gone. What remains is their legacy of love and caring. That is what we have to learn from their lives and their work.

After the funerals, for the immediate families, the reality sinks in slowly. They know life has to go on. The rest of the family has to be looked after and bills have to be paid. Days go by, weeks go by, and months go by.

Gulshan's six children have grown and settled in life except for Rozmin who has multiple sclerosis. She is in a group home in Edmonton. Rozmin's two daughters are now adults. Mansur's children are now adults. His son, Aleem, is now a physician and is in the residency program in internal medicine at Foothills Hospital in Calgary and Rehana is finishing a degree in education at University of Calgary.

Gulshan Dharamshi (1935-1996)
Mansur Bharwani (1948-1984)
Dr. Ivan Witt (1952-2001)

11

Bald is beautiful and shiny is sexy

There is one thing about baldness—it's neat.

~ Don Herold

Mirror, mirror on the wall, who's most anxious of us all?
Probably, yours truly!
These were the first two sentences of my column that I wrote before I went bald. Yes, it happened on Friday May 30, 2003. The Canadian Cancer Society was having its annual fundraising event called *Relay for Life* at Kin Coulee Park in Medicine Hat, Alberta.

The *Relay for Life* is an event that celebrates survival, pays tribute to the lives of loved ones and it is a night of fun, friendship and fundraising to beat cancer.

The question I posed to the readers of my column and through this book to you is this: What do you think of baldness? Is baldness beautiful, balderdash or just neat?

Hair has many useful functions. It protects our skin from many external elements. In our society, it has a significant psychosocial importance. But hair loss is a common problem, and it can be a distressing symptom of illness or treatment.

We are born with approximately 100,000 hair follicles on the scalp. They are predetermined to grow long, thick hair. The rest of the body has other hair follicles which are predetermined to grow short, fine, and less pigmented hair. Growth of hair is regulated by complex messages which are not well understood.

What causes hair loss?

There is hereditary thinning of the hair induced by androgens in genetically susceptible men and women. Thinning of the hair begins between the ages of 12 and 40 years in both sexes, and approximately half the population expresses this trait to some degree before the age of 50, says an article in the *New England Journal of Medicine* (NEJM).

There are many other reasons for hair loss as well, usually transient shedding of hair is associated with drugs, fever, hormonal abnormalities, pregnancy, anemia and malnutrition.

For cancer patients, it is usually chemotherapy. Chemotherapy consists of drugs to kill cancer cells. The drugs are useful in patients who have cancer at more than one site. The disadvantage is all cancer cells may not be susceptible to these drugs and chemotherapy kills some normal and healthy cells as well.

Chemotherapy entails lengthy treatments with side-effects such as hair loss, nausea, vomiting, diarrhea, depression and weakening of the body's immune system.

Shiny is sexy? Balderdash.

This was the headline to a news item in the *National Post* in November 2000. A survey of 1,502 Canadians discovered a significant number of males and females believed it was harder for a balding man to find a partner, a good job or respect in society.

The survey by the Canadian Hair Research Foundation found 60 per cent of women prefer men with hair and the number rises to 74 per cent among respondents aged 18 to 24. However, 70 per cent of men surveyed – with or without hair – reported to be involved in sexual relationships. So in reality, it may not be too hard for a bald individual to find a partner.

There is a website called *Bald R Us* (http://www.baldrus.com). The site is designed for "those who believe that God made a few perfect heads and on the rest He put hair." In the first year of operation the site attracted 10,000 members who are proud of their baldness. It is not unusual for the website to celebrate Yul Brynner's birthday in July to honour his magnificent shaved dome and for being the iconoclast of baldness. Brynner was born in Sakhalin, Russia on July 11, 1915.

In my family, my mom was shocked to hear I was getting my head shaved. My wife was speechless. My children thought it was funny. But they were proud this was for a good cause.

In my mind the question was: Did God give me a perfect head? I don't know what others think but I am happy with what I have been blessed with.

But people keep asking me, "Why did you do it?"

I believe, there is usually more than one reason why a person will do something different than what he or she is used to doing. My case was no different.

I have been raising funds for the Cancer Society for many years. But lately I had found it difficult and embarrassing to ask the same generous people to donate for the same cause each year. In a small city such as Medicine Hat, same people are asked to donate money to a variety of charities each year. I am sure some people do get tired of being asked so often. So, I thought getting my head shaved would be a dramatic way to do something different and draw people's attention.

I also did this for my cancer patients. Over the years, I have looked after many cancer patients. They have been young and they have been old, and they have come from all walks of life. There is hardly a family that has not been affected by cancer.

I am no exception. In 1996, my sister Gulshan was diagnosed with pancreatic cancer. She died within three months of diagnosis. She was young at 60. She was beginning to plan her life into retirement and travel with her husband when she was told to make plans for the last journey.

The final reason why I decided to have my head shaved for the Cancer Society was to start Docs for Cancer, similar to Cops for Cancer. Cops for Cancer is an annual event in which my son, Hussein, took part in 1997 when he was 10 years old. I hope Docs for Cancer will be embraced by physicians to raise funds for the Cancer Society.

But individual priorities vary a lot. We have our own causes to advance. We do what we can for what we believe in. There are millions of unsung heroes in this world who do charity work in a quiet way. They make this world a better place to live in, with or without being bald.

God made a few perfect heads and on the rest He put hair!
~ Bald R Us Website

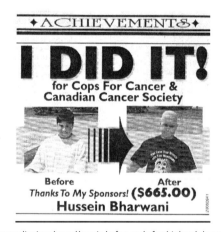

1997 – This newspaper clipping shows Hussein before and after his head shave for Cops for Cancer.

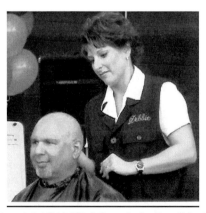

2003 – This picture shows hairstylist Debbie Bullman shaving Noorali's head for Docs for Cancer.

12

⁂

The joy of skiing

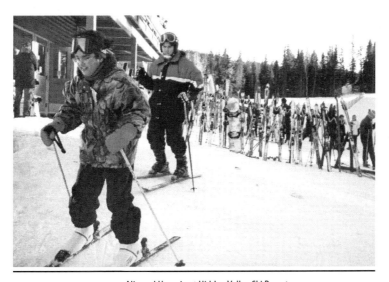

1997 – Alia and Hussein at Hidden Valley Ski Resort
in Cypress Hills Provincial Park, Elkwater, Alberta.

There's an intrinsic value in doing something
without being the best at it.
~ Susie Gephardt

Let's talk about skiing.

I had never skied in my life. At the ripe age of 50, I started taking ski lessons when my son, Hussein, joined the Nancy Green program at the Hidden Valley Ski Resort in Cypress Hills Provincial Park, Elkwater, Alberta. It is a 40 minute drive from Medicine Hat. It is the "Snoasis of the Prairie." It is interesting to note the township of Elkwater and the township of Banff are at the same elevation.

Hussein has been a fast learner. He has now moved on to snowboarding. I am still struggling with the green runs!

My daughter, Alia, likes to ski, but her enthusiasm fluctuates. My wife, Sabiya, feels that she would be a better family cheerleader rather than a skier. She supplies us with hot chocolate, lunch and snack during breaks. Not a bad deal!

Learning to ski has not been easy for me. My progress has been slow but steady. I have fear of heights and speed. I also have a fear of injury. As a surgeon, I don't want to break my wrist or ankle and be out of commission for several months. But I was determined to learn and be with my family so I have persevered.

I had never seen snow while growing up in Tanzania except in pictures of Mount Kilimanjaro. Kilimanjaro is famous for its snow-capped peak. But I never got a chance to get there. In any case, there is no skiing on Mount Kilimanjaro.

I invested a lot of money and time in taking lessons at the Hidden Valley Ski Resort, at the Canada Olympic Park in Calgary and at Sunshine Village in Banff, Alberta. Many young instructors and friends have helped me in my endeavor.

Each year by October, I look forward to winter, snow and skiing. I find skiing very relaxing and good for stress relief. I have learned to dress for winter (layers!) and I find winter months go by pretty fast.

Generally speaking, skiers are happy people. Unlike golfers, skiers are always smiling and are ecstatic when they come flying down the hills or mountains. Skiers don't shout fore and you don't hear anybody swear, unless they take a tumble!

Skiers are not rushing or pushing you to keep moving. They don't phone the clubhouse because of slow play. There is no marshal in a red power cart chasing you around the ski hills. Instead, you see helpful ski patrols and instructors.

Skiers don't slice or hook. They just fall flat on their back or front. Beginners and experienced skiers have fun together. Good skiers don't look down on beginners or show any signs of arrogance. In fact, they are willing to share their experience. It is like a big happy family.

Do you know what happens to a golfer after he dies? St. Peter sends him straight to heaven because he has suffered enough on the golf course!

For skiers, heaven is in the mountains and the ski hills. Skiers don't have to worry about life after death. It is heavenly all the way!

Hidden Valley is our jewel in the middle of the Prairies. It is in the beautiful evergreen forests of the Cypress Hills Provincial Park. It has family oriented ski hills which have done a lot for me and my family and for hundreds of other families who use it. I have met people from Medicine Hat, Brooks, Taber, Oyen, and from several places in Saskatchewan and sometimes Montana at the ski hill.

Hidden Valley has an elevation of 1,400 m (4,594 ft.) with annual snowfall of 210 cm (seven feet). The longest run is two kilometers and vertical drop of 200 m. (656 ft.).

Hidden Valley instructors have taught and continue to teach thousands of children and adults how to ski and snowboard, including an aging late bloomer like me!

During weekdays, it is busy with school trips coming from different places. It saves these children the expense of travelling to the mountains.

Winter can be very depressing because most activities are indoors. Hidden Valley is God's gift to the people of this area for fresh air and sunshine.

Our population is increasing and it is time we see some more development at Hidden Valley. I think it needs another chair lift to service the Hidden Valley run where the T-bar is. Right now this run is underutilized as many skiers are reluctant to use the T-bar.

Come to think of it, 30 years ago, there was only a toboggan hill about half a mile south of Hidden Valley used by local residents. Then there was a rope tow at the same site and the beginning of skiing in this area. In 1967, a T-bar was installed with several runs.

In 1981, Dave Fischer, father of the current owner, Kevin Fischer, took over the operation and planning for the area. In 1987, at the beginning of the re-development, the area was renamed Hidden Valley.

The re-development was undertaken by the Government of Alberta. It included a quad chair, two handle tows, a full-service day lodge, snowmaking system, run development and re-contouring of the entire base area. The combined lift capacity is 2,400 skiers per hour.

There are ambitious plans to enhance the Cypress Hills Ski facility by increasing snowmaking capability, installing a second chair lift to service the Hidden Valley run where the current T-bar is, and making additions to the existing day lodge facility.

Now Alberta's budget is balanced and we are in surplus, it is time for the government to re-invest in this project which promotes a healthy lifestyle. It will fit quite well with the government's campaign to promote Healthy U.

The investment will bring in more tourists and businesses for the local communities. It will help instill lifelong healthy skills in our children, who will pass them on to their children and grandchildren. It is an investment of immense long-term healthy benefits for generations to come.

Well, where are my skis?

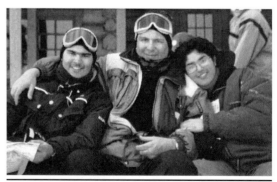

2001 – Hussein, Noorali and Alia on a ski trip to Sunshine Village near Banff in Alberta.

13

Golf is a wacky game

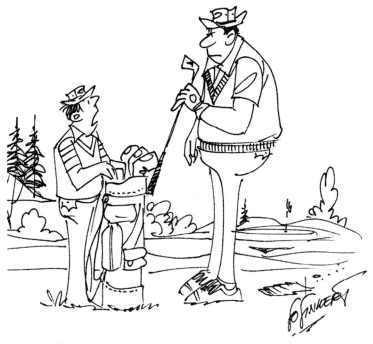

"The way I see it doctor, your problem is iron deficiency!"

The Medical Post

From the Medical Post

"Golf is not about shooting a number, it's an opportunity to live well," says Golf Guru in the *Golf Digest*. "Golf is a good walk spoiled," says Mark Twain (1835-1910). What do you think?

Like everything else in my life, I took up golf late. I was over 40 years old. I was always in a hurry to play and get back to work or home. Those days I used to work round the clock. Being on-call and doing lots of elective and emergency surgeries did not help. There was no time to relax. Besides, many people believe, due to the nature of the golf game (stop and go), walking while golfing is not counted as exercise. But an article in *Golf Digest* changed my thinking. It said golfing and walking is healthy.

An average player covers eight kilometers (five miles) or more during each 18-hole round. The article quotes a Swedish study that examined the physiological demands placed on middle-age golfers who walk the course. The researchers found that despite the short walking intervals, the golfers' exercise intensity ranged from 40 to 70 per cent of maximum aerobic power. They calculated that four hours of activity on a golf course is comparable to a 45-minute fitness class.

While golfing, you can burn 250 to 500 calories an hour. A *Golf Digest* study showed a golfer who walks 18 holes while carrying his bag travels an average of 9.4 km (5.9 miles) and burns 1,811 calories. A rider with no cart path restrictions, surprisingly, travels an average of 3.7 km (2.3 miles) and burns 859 calories.

Golf is not good for building stamina. But it is good for flexibility and has a small effect on building strength.

There is a study done by a cardiologist, Dr. Edward A. Palank, which looks at the effect of walking on cholesterol levels. The study found a group of middle-aged men who played golf three times a week for four months had LDL (bad cholesterol) levels decrease significantly compared to controls. There was no change in the HDL (good cholesterol) level.

Walking has many health benefits, whether you walk a golf course, a sidewalk, a park or a treadmill in the warmth of your basement. It will keep you fit without the risk of serious injury. It is a very natural form of exercise and anyone can do it.

Walking improves cardio-vascular fitness, lowers cholesterol levels and blood pressure. Walking burns calories, improves muscle tone, relieves tension, improves digestion and makes one feel good about one's self. It also helps prevent osteoporosis.

Most golfers are very enthusiastic about their sport. Almost nothing can stop a golfer from playing unless there is thunder and lightning. It is the challenge and the love of the outdoors (not the ball!) which gets the best and the worst out of a golfer.

A survey by *Golf Digest* asked, "Would you give up sex with your spouse to become a member at Augusta National?" Thirty per cent said "yes." I don't know the marital status of those who said "yes," but it is good to know that the majority of golfers have their priorities in the right place!

But golf is not all fun. Golf is one of the most difficult, frustrating and unpredictable games. Patience and perseverance do help if you are able to be patient and persevere.

Each golfing season starts with the golfer's desire to cut his handicap by a reasonable number. Unfortunately, this fails. It has been shown even among the most dedicated players only 25 per cent will improve their handicap index by at least one stroke during a 12-month period.

At the request of *Golf Digest*, the U.S. Golf Association studied the handicap indexes of more than 1.1-million golfers from 2002 to 2003 and found that only two per cent of players improved by five strokes or more during that 12-month span. The biggest shocker: 50 per cent of players got worse!

It is said golf mimics life. During a round of golf, a golfer faces so many challenges (called hazards) that after playing 18 holes the golfer is usually left frustrated.

A good golfer needs a good swing. The mechanics of a good swing have been thoroughly studied, but very few can duplicate them.

The ball, with multiple dimples, is supposed to fly like a bird and provide good distance. They are expensive to buy. So, most golfers end up buying cheap "experienced" balls because who wants to throw away money in the multiple ponds and creeks they call hazards!

Golfers are like farmers. An accurate weather forecast is important for them. Playing in the wind and rain is no fun. Sometime golfers do get lucky with sunny days and no wind. Then they never stop talking about it!

Golfers have to worry and cope with the mosquitoes and West Nile virus. Using a mosquito repellent containing DEET is a good idea. Sunny days also increase the risk of skin cancer. The Canadian Dermatology Association recommends using a sunscreen with a sun protection factor (SPF) of between 30 and 60.

Dehydration and fatigue can be dangerous. Golfers have to drink plenty of water. In 2002, a 15-year-old boy in Phoenix contracted Norwalk virus (he subsequently died) from a golf course water cooler. Eighty other golfers fell ill. The Canadian National Golf Course Owners Association had recommended its 2,300 member courses remove all coolers. But some golf courses still have them.

Golfers do get hungry. It is good to pack snacks which do not contain refined flour, sugar or trans fats (they can clog arteries). Try nuts, seeds, fruits and low-carbohydrate bars.

Golf is fun if you like it and have reasonable expectations. As somebody said, the world of golf has loads of weird terms, wild rules and wacky practices. Either you love it or you hate it. There is no fun if you are sitting on the fence. Then you might as well be a politician!

Well, when is my next tee time?

Once upon a time, a guy asked a girl, "Will you marry me?"
The girl said, "No." And the guy played a lot of golf
and lived happily ever after. The End.
~ World's shortest fairy tale from *Golf Digest*

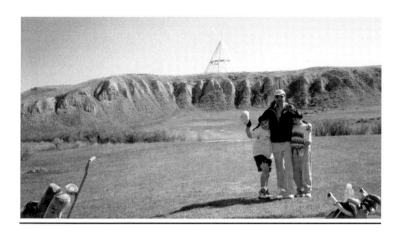

1997 – Hussein, Noorali and Alia at Paradise Valley Golf Course in Medicine Hat, Alberta. The world's tallest teepee in the background.

14

❊

Confessions of a snorer!

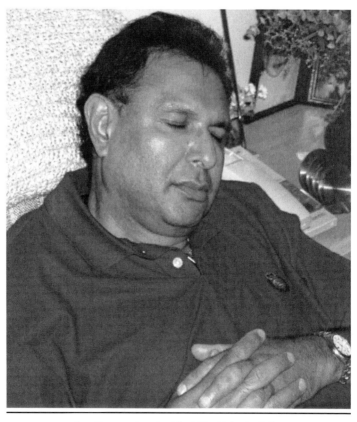

1997 – Noorali on a snoring trip while visiting his brother in Vancouver.

Do you snore?

I do!

Probably everyone does.

Then why do I feel so guilty about it?

One morning, I read the local newspaper and keep quiet. My daughter, Alia, looks at the paper and says, "Mom, did you read this? It says: Laugh and the world laughs with you, snore and you sleep alone."

My wife, Sabiya, looks at me and smiles.

Why? Because I snore.

I have no trouble sleeping. During my surgical residency days, I would go off to sleep while assisting in the operating room on a long case because I could hardly see what I was doing. The surgeon's shoulder was always in my way!

One afternoon, after a busy night on call, I dozed off in the Royal Alexandra Hospital library in Edmonton. My loud snoring not only woke me up, but when I opened my eyes, there were about 15 students and residents staring at me.

I have become so self-conscious of my snoring that I am afraid to doze off in public. Travelling by plane is a good example. Sharing a hotel room with my friends and family is a nightmare. Sitting through all-day meetings or seminars can be taxing if I cannot take a catnap. If somebody in my family does not get a good night's sleep they blame it on me and my snoring. When it comes to snoring even walls have ears!

I just blame my snoring on my genes. My father used to snore. My mother still snores. Her snoring does not bother me – probably I snore louder than her but her snoring does bother others. Some of my brothers and sisters snore.

My wife has tried all the tricks on me: nudging me to turn on my side, pinching my nose, even putting a pillow on my face. That is when I saw danger. So now I sleep with only one pillow. Why have a spare one and invite trouble!

You would think that all this anxiety would give me sleepless nights. No. When I put my head on the pillow, I am gone. And my wife says the "engine" starts right away.

Snoring is a significant social problem. Approximately 20 per cent of all adults – including nearly 50 per cent of those over 60 years of age – are chronic snorers. Snoring is part of the sleep-related breathing disorders called "sleep disordered breathing." Snoring occurs because of sleep-induced airway obstruction.

Most snorers have sleep apnea as well. Normally, breathing is regular. In sleep apnea there is an interruption in breathing during sleep.

Sleep apnea may be central, that is due to instability of the feedback system that regulates breathing. Or sleep apnea may be obstructive, due to recurrent obstruction of the upper airway. Or it can be mixed, central followed by obstructive.

Obstructive sleep apnea affects 2 per cent of women and 4 per cent of men. It is a condition of middle-aged adults.

A typical individual with obstructive sleep apnea starts snoring shortly after going to sleep. The snoring proceeds at a regular pace for a period of time, often becoming louder, but is then interrupted by a long silent period during which no breathing is taking place (apnea). The apnea is then interrupted by a loud snort and gasp and the snoring returns to its regular pace. This behaviour may recur repetitively and frequently throughout the night.

Obstructive sleep apnea causes frequent night awakening, feeling of tiredness in the morning, abnormal daytime sleepiness, headaches, memory loss, poor judgment, personality changes and lethargy. It may also raise the blood pressure.

Who suffers from obstructive sleep apnea?

Obstructive sleep apnea occurs most frequently in obese middle-aged men. Contributing factors may include use of alcohol or sedatives before sleep, anatomically narrowed airways, and massively enlarged tonsils and adenoids. Genetic and environmental factors may also adversely affect airway size. The condition may run in some families.

Diagnosis of sleep apnea is made by sleep studies. Sleep study should be strongly considered for two groups of patients: those who habitually snore and report daytime sleepiness, and those who habitually snore and have observed apnea (regardless of daytime symptoms).

Are there any medical or physical side effects to obstructive sleep apnea?

Once upon a time, sleep apnea was thought to imply poor prognosis. It was thought to arise from the diseases of the brain and heart. It is now known that periodic breathing generally occurs during sleep, and that it may occur in healthy persons.

During periodic breathing, there is change in the partial pressure of carbon dioxide and oxygen in the blood and this result in the fluctuation of heart rate (with irregular rhythm) and blood pressure and in the autonomic nervous system. Heart failure, heart attack and stroke are other likely complications.

Chronic sleep deprivation caused by sleep apnea increases the risk of motor vehicle collisions. The collision rate for such patients has been reported to be seven times that of the general driving population.

Does obstructive sleep apnea really damage our health?

In 1997, a review article in the *British Medical Journal* evaluated all studies published between 1966 and 1995 on the association between obstructive sleep apnea and mortality and morbidity, and on the efficacy of nasal continuous positive airways pressure. The authors concluded there was limited evidence of increased mortality or morbidity in patients with obstructive sleep apnea.

They also concluded the evidence linking the condition to cardiac irregular rhythm, coronary artery disease, heart failure, high blood pressure, pulmonary hypertension, stroke, and automobile collisions was conflicting and inconclusive. They concluded that there was insufficient data to determine its effect on quality of life, morbidity or mortality.

In 2005, an observational study, published in the *New England Journal of Medicine*, found that patients who experienced five or more apneic episodes per hour were twice as likely to have a stroke or die in the next three years. Worsening sleep apnea was associated with increased risk.

So who is right?

Is there a need to do anything about snoring and obstructive sleep apnea?

It is important to consult your physician and let him or her assess your risk factors for heart and lung disease and then decide about the management of sleep apnea. In general I would suggest the following:

Treatment of snoring is required if a person snores to the extent that the marital relationship may be threatened. Then you may snore alone in the basement of your house or few miles away in an isolated barn! Or get help!

Treatment is also required if the sleep disorder affects daytime sleepiness and alters the function of the heart and the lungs.

The goals of treatment are to abolish snoring and eliminate disruption of sleep due to upper-airway obstruction. This will establish an adequate oxygen level in the blood and adequate ventilation system.

Treatment strategies are divided into three general categories:
- Behavioural modification
- Medical treatment
- Surgical treatment

Counseling for behavioural changes includes losing weight, avoidance of alcohol and sedatives. Most patients snore sleeping on their back. These patients should be asked to train themselves to sleep exclusively on their side.

Medical management of sleep apnea revolves around positive airway pressure (PAP), dental appliance and medications. There is no good medication to help sleep apnea. Sometimes oxygen therapy helps.

The positive airway pressure is delivered through a mask to be worn when asleep. The machine that creates PAP weighs two kilograms.

The cost of the system may run into a couple of thousand dollars. PAP keeps the upper airway open during sleep. Compliance of this method of treatment is not 100 per cent. One study demonstrated 46 per cent of patients used PAP for more than four hours per night for more than 70 per cent of the observed nights. Some people may find the system difficult to use. Others have adapted quite nicely. Some studies have shown improved survival in patients who use PAP.

Oral appliance has been promoted as a useful alternative to PAP. There are varieties of appliances. The appliances are worn only during sleep and are generally well tolerated. Not all patients have clinically proven response. It is considered as a second line of treatment compared to PAP.

Surgical treatment for snoring and obstructive sleep apnea has become quite popular recently, probably due to the inconvenience of PAP and oral appliance. Several surgical procedures are available, each one with advantages and disadvantages. These procedures are done by otolaryngologists (specialists in ear, nose and throat surgeries).

Not all snorers require major surgery involving the palate. Fixing simple problems in the nose and throat can make a significant difference. Major surgical procedures involving the palate and pharynx is successful in abolishing snoring in about two thirds of selected patients. That means in one-third of the patients the surgical treatment will fail. There is a fair amount of pain for the first few days after surgery.

There isn't one good solution to the problem of snoring and obstructive sleep apnea. The decision is based on personal need. If you don't want to snort with the pigs in the barn then seek help. See your doctor and he will send you for sleep study and decide on what options will best fit your needs.

But before you rush for surgery, think of trying something simple such as exercise, weight loss, decreased alcohol consumption, smoking cessation, altered sleeping position, PAP and dental or nasal appliances.

Dr. Noorali Bharwani

Good luck. Until then, happy snoring!

> *Life is a dream; when we sleep we are awake,*
> *and when awake we sleep.*
> ~ Michel de Montaigne (1533-1592)

15

The art of being kind

So many gods, so many creeds,
So many paths that wind and wind,
While just the art of being kind
Is all the sad world needs.
~ Ella Wheeler Wilcox (1855-1919)

The door bell rings. It's Saturday, 8 a.m. It's a Thanksgiving weekend. A gentleman stands at the door and hands over an item which we had lost recently. He found it and wanted to make sure we get it before the holiday weekend.

This gentleman, we shall call him Sean, was leaving town for the long weekend. But his thoughts and concerns were with our family. He wanted the item delivered to our house personally. We were very impressed and touched by Sean's total selfless gesture.

Through my newspaper column I expressed my family's gratitude to Sean for his kindness, thoughtfulness and generosity in stopping by at our house. He made our Thanksgiving weekend very special, it had a real meaning to it. I am sure Sean felt the same way.

This act of kindness also brought in me a sense of guilt and made me examine my own acts gone by. Have I been kind enough to make a difference in somebody's life? Is there somebody out there who feels I have been unfair or unkind? In my own heart, is there a gap between perception and reality on what kindness means?

Nobody is perfect so I must be guilty of some unkindness. We all have our share of mistakes, misjudgments and acts of stupidity. In the end the question is, do we really care about others to make a difference in their lives?

Sir Rabindranath Tagore (1861-1941) said, "Men are cruel, but man is kind." We just have to look at the world around us. On one hand there is death and destruction and on the other hand there is kindness and generosity. It is hard to believe men can be so cruel and still be so kind.

As a physician, the obligation of being kind is even more important. The Canadian Medical Association's Code of Ethics says that a physician's ethic of service is characterized by the values of:

- compassion,
- beneficence (quality of being kind, charitable, or beneficial),
- nonmaleficence (do no harm),
- respect for persons, and
- justice.

Each day and during a physician's lifetime of practice, he will see many patients and do numerous tests and procedures. By the law of averages, somebody is going to have complications and somebody is going to be unhappy. Somebody is going to feel that a physician is uncaring and unkind. It is impossible to satisfy everybody.

Does that mean we give up on being kind? No. An act of kindness does not always end in a win-win situation, but the majority of the time it should and it does. Sean's act of kindness is one example, and that is very encouraging. Just the art of being kind is all the sad world needs!

Thank you, Sean! Keep up the good work.

16

Fighting mosquitoes

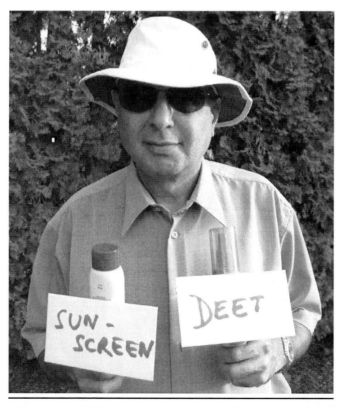

Do not lower your guard. When you are outdoors, protect yourself against the damaging effects of sunrays and mosquito bites with wide-brimmed hat, sunglasses, sunscreen and DEET.

I have been fighting mosquitoes all my life.

It all started in Musoma, Tanzania where I was born and raised. There was no electricity and no telephone. The radio worked on an old-fashioned car battery which needed to be charged every couple of days. The drinking water had to be boiled first. Malaria-infested mosquitoes were everywhere.

Although much has changed in Africa now, malaria continues to be a dreaded illness. It kills an African child every 30 seconds. Being attacked by mosquitoes was like being attacked by the birds in Hitchcock's famous movie!

In Musoma, every evening, all the rooms in the house had to be sprayed with Dichlorodiphenyltrichloroethane (DDT); a colorless contact insecticide. DDT is toxic to humans and animals when swallowed or absorbed through the skin. Each night, at bed time, we had to take a pill called Paludrin, as a prophylaxis against malaria.

We could not sleep at night without a mosquito net. Quite often a mosquito would get inside the net and buzz all night. You would be lucky if you did not get your blood sucked that night.

Doing homework in the evenings was a nightmare. Malaria-infested mosquitoes come out after dark to attack. The kerosene-lit lamps would attract all kinds of bugs. DDT was used generously.

Then I went to India for higher education. The mosquito problem was the same. Mosquito nets had to be used, but there was no fear of malaria as India was free from that illness.

Then I spent several years in the United Kingdom. I don't remember fighting mosquitoes there. It was always cold and damp. Mosquitoes are smart. They don't like cold weather.

In Canada, I did not find mosquitoes a menace until I started golfing. I remember we used to complain about sand flies. Now we talk only about mosquitoes.

I don't like mosquitoes. I am allergic to their bites. When I go golfing, I apply a good layer of sunscreen. Then I generously spray DEET (N,N-Diethyl-meta-Toluamide) to the exposed areas of my body and my clothes. DEET is a colourless, oily liquid, $C_{12}H_{17}NO$,

that has a mild odour and is used as an insect repellent.
The chemicals immediately change my body odour. The odour
is tolerable when I am on the golf course and my friends probably
don't care how I smell. But when I come home, I am not touchable,
not huggable, nor kissable. In spite of a thorough shower, my body
odour is chemically compromised for 12 to 24 hours.

In spite of all the precautions, I still end up getting at least three
to five mosquito bites. They itch and burn after a shower. Then I
apply After Bite to control the itching. That leaves its own smell on
my body. I wonder how much damage these chemicals have caused
and continue to cause to my skin and some important organs of my
anatomy.

According to World Health Organization website, DDT has now
been banned from agricultural use. Maybe I should have been a
vegetable! But DDT still has an important role to play in saving lives
and reducing the burden of malaria in some of the world's poorest
countries. Eventually, the plan is to eliminate the production and use
of DDT.

Malaria is a life-threatening parasitic disease transmitted by
mosquitoes. Today approximately 40 per cent of the world's
population, mostly those living in the world's poorest countries, is at
risk of malaria. It causes more than 300-million acute illnesses and at
least one-million deaths a year.

Africa is also the source of West Nile virus. It was first isolated
in 1937 from the blood of a patient on the West Nile province of
Uganda. The man had a fever. Initially, the outbreaks of the disease
were few. But in the last 10 years the numbers have increased.

In North America, the virus was first detected in 1999. It was in
New York. From there it was exported to Ontario. In 2003, about
400 people in Ontario became infected with the virus. At least 19
people have died.

Most cases of West Nile virus are mild and self-resolving. But one
per cent of cases get infection in the nervous system.

As I have learned over the years, mosquitoes are dangerous.

If you want to enjoy the fresh air and the outdoors then learn to protect yourself. I take no chances. Besides, I react quite badly to the mosquito bites. Ouch!

"More than 40 per cent of the world's population is at risk of malaria, and more than a million people die of it each year. Malaria kills a child every 30 seconds: 90 per cent of people who die from malaria are children not yet five years of age, and most (90 per cent) of these deaths take place in sub-Saharan Africa."

~ The Canadian Medical Association Journal, January 17, 2006

17

Finding the centre of consciousness

No one can carry you to the mountain top.
You can be guided, but eventually you must climb to the peak
yourself to achieve complete mastery.
~ Martin and Marian Jerry in *Sutras of the Inner Teacher*

Do you know what a centre of consciousness is? Have you ever thought of finding one? Once you find it, what do you do with it? What has yoga and meditation to do with the centre of consciousness?

Answers to these and many other questions can be found in a book titled *Sutras of the Inner Teacher– The Yoga of the Centre of Consciousness* (2M Communications, Canmore, Canada). It is written by Drs. Martin and Marian Jerry, physician-scientist and clinical psychologist respectively.

The Jerrys are now retired and live in Canmore, Alberta.

During the Family Day (March 21, 2005) long week-end, I decided to visit Canmore. I wanted to ski with my friends and to pay my respects to my mentor, the man who gave me a start in Canada.

That mentor happens to be Dr. Martin Jerry. I also had a selfish reason to visit him and his lovely wife. I wanted to discuss and get advice on a couple of projects I was working on, including the plans for this book.

I first met Martin Jerry when I came to visit my parents in Calgary in the summer of 1979. I had finished my surgical training in Britain and was looking for a research fellowship in Canada.

Jerry was then Professor of Medicine at the University of Calgary and Director of the Oncology Research Group of what later was to become Tom Baker Cancer Centre.

Jerry told me that he was looking for a research fellow in cancer immunology and the funding from the National Cancer Institute of Canada (NCIC) was already in place. After an interview and after completing other formalities he offered me the position that carried NCIC fellowship stipend of $1,000 per month.

I was single. At the age of 34, I lived with my parents like a student, made some sacrifices and survived. I spent two years with Jerry's group. I remember Jerry as an outstanding teacher, clinician, researcher and mentor who took good care of me and all those who worked under his stewardship. I also had the pleasure of knowing his wonderful wife, Marian, and their two sons, Paul and Mark.

In fact Paul Jerry is a chartered psychologist in Medicine Hat. What a coincidence.

Over the years I have been in touch with the Jerrys. I keep them informed on the progress I make in life. I feel the man who gave me a start in Canada should know how I am doing. I am also fascinated with their book. I would like to find my centre of consciousness, find spiritual enlightenment and take care of my fears and phobias. Is yoga and meditation the answer?

I believe so. Only time will tell whether I have the discipline to achieve that spiritual enlightenment. The Jerrys' book says, "No one can carry you to the mountain top. You can be guided, but eventually you must climb to the peak yourself to achieve complete mastery."

The book is a good guide, and the visit to Canmore was very enriching. We talked about the past, the present and the future. I got the advice I needed to keep my projects on the right track and learnt again that there are kind and caring people in this world who do make a difference in a very private and quiet way. For that I am thankful. I pray for their good health and happy retirement.

19

Do no harm

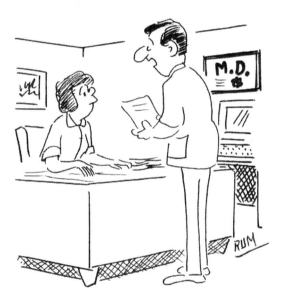

"If it's true that you learn from your mistakes,
then you must be one of the smartest persons in the city."

The Medical Post, December 7, 1997

"No one cares how much you know
until they know how much you care."
~ Theodore Roosevelt

What is the difference between God and a doctor? God does not think he is a doctor!

You have heard this joke before. But it is not funny when you are a patient and your doctor thinks he is God, he knows it all and he can do no wrong. What you want to know is does he care?

Life without mistakes is impossible. In medicine we deal with people. We have to offer them a better and healthier life which is pain free and comfortable. This is why patient safety is so important. Any treatment offered to a patient should improve his or her life. But errors in medicine do occur. From time to time diagnoses will be missed and complications from treatment will occur. That is why it is said that to err is human.

A report released in the U.S. in 2004 says medical errors kill about 100,000 Americans each year. The chairman of the 19-member panel that issued the report says, "These stunningly high rates of medical errors resulting in deaths, permanent disability, and unnecessary suffering are simply unacceptable in a medical system that promises first to 'do no harm'."

An editorial in the *British Medical Journal* says studies in Australia, Israel, the United Kingdom and elsewhere, suggest levels of error and hazard in patient care that are no lower than in America. Canada is not immune to the problem.

Should health-care professionals be superhuman?

No. But the public and the politicians expect them to be. After all, they are highly trained individuals.

John Hubbard, in a book called *Measuring Medical Education*, says two types of physicians make mistakes – a *shotgunner*, who prescribes and does procedures without adequate information and indications, and a *timid soul*, who makes diagnoses without adequate information.

But there are other reasons for errors as well which people fail to appreciate. Overworked and underpaid workers, inadequate resources, manpower shortages, political interference and personal and family stress do not provide a healthy environment for error-free practice.

Is there a mechanism to prevent errors in medicine?

Yes, the American report condemns the current fragmented system of handling medical mistakes, which relies on a combination of peer review, federal and state regulation, malpractice lawsuits, and evaluations by professional bodies. The panel suggests mandatory reporting and public disclosure of serious medical errors.

In my view, there are five ways to prevent medical errors:

1. Make sure the patient understands you care

2. Do not do anything you are not comfortable with

3. Communicate with the patient using simple language

4. Know your strengths and weaknesses

5. Learn to say "I don't know."

Physicians who communicate well with patients and their families do better when things do not go according to plan. Unfortunately, not all physicians have good communication skills, especially when it comes to bereaved family members.

"A physician's responsibility for the care of a patient does not end when the patient dies. There is one final responsibility: to help the bereaved family members. A letter of condolence can contribute to the healing of bereaved family and help achieve closure in the relationship between the physician and the patient's family," says an article in the *New England Journal of Medicine (NEJM)*.

How often do we, the physicians, do this? Hardly ever. Well, I shouldn't say that. There is always somebody somewhere who does special things for people he cares about. Let me tell you about my own practice and how things have evolved over the years. This is not only about bereavement. It is also about caring and making patients feel good.

Let me start with an example. A patient whom I had known for many years was hospitalized with complications from a long-standing illness. I was not directly involved in her care, but I knew she was in the hospital. From time to time, I dropped in to say hello, hold her hand and spend a few minutes talking about things in general. A few days later, she died. I received a thank you card from the family for having taken care of her in the past and was told how much my visits and services were appreciated by the patient and the family. I asked my receptionist to give me her file so I could call the family and give my condolences. The file lay on my desk for two weeks and I never got around to phoning.

This is in complete contrast to what I used to do when I started my practice in Medicine Hat in 1985. I had no children, my practice was not that busy and I had plenty of time to spend with my patients and their families.

I used to do my ward rounds twice a day. Morning rounds are usually "quickies," as we are rushing to the office or to the operating room. Evening rounds allowed me to sit with my patients and learn more about their illness and family. Occasionally, I sent flowers to patients who had major surgery. Some times my wife visited them in the hospital.

Those days, on weekends, I used to take my five-year-old son, Hussein, to meet my patients. We had a white coat made for him and he would carry his plastic stethoscope in his pocket. Many of my patients still remember this. Even now they ask me how my little boy is doing. Of course now he is an adult. A few years later I started taking my daughter as well. Weekends were a good time to spend a little extra time with my patients. Patients remember those extra visits and extra time you spend with them more than what you do for them medically and surgically. Kindness and caring usually provoke no complications!

As I got busy with my practice and my family, the evening rounds occurred only if a patient was sick and needed another visit to check his or her progress. The desire to rush home and play with my kids was irresistible after a long day in the hospital and office.

In my practice I don't remember having written a letter of condolence to bereaving family members. Occasionally, I have phoned. Contact with the patients in hospital is now to a minimum. Most patients are discharged the same day or day after surgery. Due to long waiting lists, the pressure to see more patients in the office does not allow too much time to talk about other things. As a specialist, it is hard to know my patients more than what they come to see me for. That old style family physician type of relationship is hard to establish.

According to the *NEJM* article, in 19th century America the process of grieving was detailed and elaborate. The doctor's letter of condolence was an accepted responsibility and an important part of the support offered to the bereaved. But today, the pattern of mourning has changed and has become much abbreviated. We forget that sometimes people need a friend rather than a doctor.

The article makes a strong point to encourage physicians to find time and write a letter to a bereaved family. It says, "Unlike expressions of condolence made by telephone or in person, a letter of condolence is a concrete gift that the recipient can and will review over and over."

In this day and age, the patient-doctor relationship has become impersonal. Now we are advancing towards the computerized paperless office, Internet medicine, tele-medicine and robotic surgery. Very soon we may not even touch a patient to make a diagnosis or provide treatment, all in the name of progress.

The primary task of a physician is to cure sometimes, to relieve often, and to comfort always.
- Author Unknown

19

A neighbour on Father's Day

In the year 2000, my neighbour died. It was unexpected. We were shocked. When I gave the tragic news to my son, his first reaction was: Dad, what will we do without Mr. Link?

That year on Father's Day, my thoughts were with Waldemar Link. Waldemar was not only a good neighbour but he was like a father to us and grandpa to our children. When we moved into his neighbourhood in 1986, Waldemar and his wife, Herta, showed us the selfless true spirit of good neighbours. Whether it was to mend a fence, check a leaking roof, build a deck, take care of the dying cedar trees or check the mail and look after the house during our holidays, they were always there.

Just a week before he died, Waldemar was there helping my son, Hussein, get a CB radio antenna cable into his room through a tiny hole in a window. If we had a problem in the house or the backyard, our first reaction was: Let us check with Mr. Link!

On Father's Day, we usually pay tribute to our real fathers. My father died in 1991. My wife's father died in 1999. Both had long and happy lives except at the end when they suffered from painful illnesses that made their lives uncomfortable. Both were lucky to live long enough to see their large families grow and settle down in life. Both were quite satisfied before their death that they had fulfilled their role in life as good fathers. They were always there when we needed them. They gave us the security and education to be independent in life.

We were lucky to have our fathers when we were growing up. But what about those young children whose fathers have been taken away from them by accident or illness? And there are fathers who have chosen to abandon their children due to reasons that are difficult to understand by third parties. Then there are fathers who have committed or continue to commit acts of terror and abuse on their children. These young children are being raised in one-parent families. Do we really understand how they feel on this day or for that matter for the rest of their lives?

What about single fathers who struggle to be good mothers as well? Does society understand and appreciate these fathers?

Most fathers try very hard to be good role models for their children. But not all fathers are paragons of virtue. We, as fathers, make mistakes like other humans. The important thing is to learn from these mistakes. Father's Day should be that day of reflection to see where we failed and where we can make a difference. What counts is the learning process of self-improvement. There are no schools for fathers to train except from what our own fathers taught us. Are we true to those teachings?

Sonora Smart Dodd started Father's Day on June 19, 1910. Sonora was raised by her father after her mother's death. Sonora's father was born in June, so the third Sunday of the month has been celebrated as Father's Day. On every Father's Day we should reflect on our past and plan a future for our children so they can carry our message to their children. Our children bear our legacy. We hope they will forgive our stupidity, learn from our mistakes and create their own standards of excellence for their children to follow.

Mr. Link and all the dads, wherever you are, have a Happy Father's Day each year for ever!

Waldemar Link (1927-1999)

20

Religion, medicine and nirvana

There is only one religion, though there are a hundred versions of it.
~ George Bernard Shaw (1856-1950)

What is religion?

To most people religion is a set of beliefs, values and practices based on the teachings of a spiritual leader. How far one takes these beliefs, values and practices depends on how one is brought up and influenced by family, friends and the environment in which he or she is raised.

I believe that religion should be a way of life. It should be about how we conduct ourselves in society, how we treat our fellow citizens, how we perceive good from bad and how we espouse our moral and ethical values.

Nobody is going to be perfect. Mistakes will be made. From time to time there will be a lapse in judgment. Our moral and ethical values will be tested and challenged. We will be judged on how we come through these tests and how we conduct ourselves in the future. That will determine where we stand in our moral and ethical values. To err is human. To get back on the right track is divine!

But things are not as straight forward as that. If a man thinks about his physical or moral state, he usually discovers that he is ill. I don't know who said that but there is some truth to it. When we look at the world within and around us we immediately realize that there is something wrong somewhere. It is a kind of illness. This illness has been present for many centuries. In order to correct this there arose, from time to time, messengers for different races of the earth, to sustain our soul and provide physical, moral and spiritual leadership.

Many use religion and spirituality to promote good health, happiness and brotherhood of man. But there are others who perpetrate violence, destruction and death in the name of religion.

This infighting among religious groups is surprising due to the "fact that no people have been discovered who do not believe in the existence and survival of human souls," says A. T. Houghton in *The World's Religions*. This book, edited by J.N.D. Anderson, provides a short factual account of the history, philosophy, and practice of seven of the great religions of the world. A study of Christianity has been excluded, as it is a well-known religion in Western countries.

Let us briefly look at the teachings of these seven great religions as described in Anderson's book: Animism, Judaism, Islam, Hinduism, Buddhism, Shintoism and Confucianism.

The book uses the term *Animism* to describe the religion and the philosophy of peoples who believe in the existence of spiritual beings. Animism is the doctrine that places the source of mental and even physical life in energy independent of, or at least distinct from, the body.

Judaism believes there is only one God in the universe, and He is the God of Israel. The book says this idea of God is to some extent similar to what the Christians and Moslems believe. Followers of all three faiths believe religion is a way of life and life needs to be cherished and not destroyed by neglect or abuse.

Islam arose to claim the allegiance of mankind about six hundred years after the appearance of Jesus Christ. Islamic beliefs are based on the Five Pillars:

1. The recital of the Creed or Kalima (There is no god but God, and Muhammad is the Prophet of God)

2. Prayer – 5 times a day
3. Fasting in the month of Ramadan
4. Zakat (tithe) or voluntary charity
5. The hajj (pilgrimage to Mecca).

Hinduism originated in India. Two important aspects of Hinduism are:

1. Triumph of good (god Vishnu) over evil (god Siva)
2. Karma – what you sow you reap. Bad and good fortune, health or sickness, poverty or riches, are all ascribed to karma.

Buddhism came into existence almost 600 years before Christ. Buddhism consists of The Four Truths:

1. The truth of suffering – suffering is omnipresent
2. Cause of suffering – desire for possession and selfish enjoyment
3. Suffering ceases, when selfish craving, lust for life, has been renounced and destroyed
4. Eightfold path that leads to the cessation of suffering – a path to perfect detachment from self-indulgence and self-mortification.

Buddhism also teaches: karma (action-reaction), impermanence (every form must die and give place to a different one), nirvana (passionless happiness).

Shintoism, the Way of the Gods, is reverence paid to the gods of Japan. Its code of moral behavior is an unwritten code that owes much to Confucius and Buddhism.

Confucius was born in 551 B.C. in China. His teaching was almost entirely concerned with man's moral conduct and his social relations. His aim was to reform the corrupt kingdom by means of moral principles of the ancient worthies.

Islam is very much in the news these days. Islam, the religion of all Muslims, was revealed to Prophet Mohamed in Arabia in the seventh century AD. Islam is an Arabic word which means "surrender." A Muslim accepts surrender to the will of Allah – Arabic for God.

The will of God (Allah) was revealed to his messenger, Mohamed, and documented in the holy book called Quran (Koran). Ramadan marks the first time the Quran was revealed to prophet Mohamed. Mohamed was the last messenger and prophet of God after Adam, Noah, Jesus and others.

Historians consider the religion of Islam as one of the outstanding phenomena of history. But Islam has no central authority (like the Vatican) to guide its followers. And there are numerous divisions and subdivisions that interpret the Quran in many different ways.

The prophet Mohamed had two sources of authority, one religious and the other secular

After the death of the prophet, two streams of thoughts split Muslims into Sunnis (the majority) and Shias (means a stream). These divisions were political rather than religious. Sunnis believed their leader ought to come from among the Meccan aristocracy and Shias felt it should remain within the prophet's blood line.

Therefore, Shias believe that after the prophet's death, divine power was transferred to Hazrat Ali, the prophet's son-in-law, as the first Imam or spiritual chief of the devout. From there on the Shias followed the guidance of hereditary Imams. Sometimes they failed to agree who the rightful Imam was, resulting in further subdivisions.

In Islam, there are no priests or monks. There is no confession of sins except to God. Cleanliness and personal hygiene are important. Prayer is a daily necessity. Wars are condemned because Islam is a religion of peace.

During the course of history, Islam has produced renowned philosophers, jurists, physicians, mathematicians, astronomers and scientists.

All religions teach the same virtues: forgiveness, kindness and generosity. I have lived in four continents and I have spent most of my adult life amongst people of different religions. I agree with Robert Burton (1577-1640), who said, "One religion is as true as another."

If one religion is as true as another then why do we need so many labels? Benjamin Disraeli (1804-1881) said, "Sensible men are all of the same religion. And what religion is that? Sensible men never tell!"

I wish there were more people sensible enough not to talk about their religious beliefs. But the current world atmosphere makes it difficult not to do that. Look at the politicians in Canada and the U.S. Religious beliefs come up for discussion all the time. Elections are fought and won on what is religiously right. It seems our values and politics are judged on the basis of our religion. There is no end to stereotyping.

I agree with Sean O'Casey (1880-1964), who said "I think we ought to have as great a regard for religion as we can, so as to keep it out of as many things as possible." To this I would add, let common sense prevail so that society can be just and kind to all people.

But every religion has its share of bigots, zealots and fanatics. This is not something new. It's been there for centuries. These people promote their brand of religious beliefs which promote divisions and hatred rather than forgiveness, kindness and generosity.

But I believe the vast majority of people (whatever their religion) use religion and spirituality to promote good health, happiness and brotherhood of man. It is used to achieve peace and tranquility in life.

Sigmund Freud (1856-1939) said, "Life as we find it is too hard for us; it entails too much pain, too many disappointments, and impossible tasks. We cannot do without palliative remedies." Unfortunately, religion is not what he had in mind when he suggested palliative remedies. In fact, he said when a man is freed of religion, he has a better chance to live a normal and wholesome life.

Some people would agree with that since every religion imposes on its followers a certain type of discipline. Some religions are more rigid than others. Many people find commonsense flexibility more attractive than dogmatic rigidity sometimes prevalent in religious surroundings.

Most sensible people carry on in life the way they feel is best for them and their families, in a quiet way, without making waves or hurting anybody's feelings. After all, one's religion should be something very personal. Many people find happiness and comfort in religious activities. And that is good. The happier you are, the healthier you feel.

Remember what George Bernard Shaw (1856-1950) said, "There is only one religion, though there are a hundred versions of it." Let us respect them all so we can do unto others what we like done to us.

Do we need religion to stay healthy and happy?

As a physician, I discuss with my patients different ways to pursue a healthy lifestyle. But I never talk about religion. I believe it is a personal and private matter.

What is interesting is a *Newsweek* poll, published some years ago, show 72 per cent of Americans would welcome a conversation with their physician about faith. The same number say they believe praying to God can cure someone, even if science says the person doesn't stand a chance.

The *Newsweek* poll says 84 per cent of Americans think praying for the sick improves their chances of recovery; 28 per cent think religion and medicine should be separate.

But what does science say?

Again there are differing opinions. The difficulty is how do you measure the power of prayer? It would be impossible to do a double blind prospective trial on the power of prayer.

The *Newsweek* article says Dr. Lynda H. Powell, an epidemiologist at Rush University Medical Center in Chicago, reviewed about 150 papers on this subject. She found while faith provides comfort in times of illness, it does not significantly slow cancer growth or improve recovery from acute illness.

There was one positive finding. People who regularly attend church have a 25 per cent reduction in mortality. They live longer than people who are not church-goers.

The *Newsweek* poll also shows 84 per cent of Americans said praying for others can have a positive effect on their recovery, and 74 per cent said that would be true even if they didn't know the patient. But this is not confirmed by scientific studies.

But whatever science says, every individual has his or her spiritual relationship with God. How we use that relationship to stay healthy depends on us. If we believe in something, then it usually works.

Should physicians prescribe religious activities to treat medical ailments—just like they prescribe antibiotics?

Why not! In an era of complementary medicine and alternative therapies, why not add religious activities to a long list of non-traditional therapies?

But the answer is not that simple. There are people who think this is not a good idea. A group of seven chaplains, representing a wide range of religions, and two biomedical researchers, have written an article in the *New England Journal of Medicine* expressing their concerns.

Polls do suggest the U.S. population is highly religious and most people believe in heaven and hell, the healing power of prayer, and the capacity of faith to aid in the recovery from disease. About 77 per cent of hospitalized patients want physicians to consider their spiritual needs in the management of their problems.

Surveys of family physicians in the U.S. strongly support the notion religious beliefs can promote healing. Nearly 30 U.S. medical schools now offer courses on religion, spirituality and health. Some physicians believe going to church promotes good health.

But the authors of the article are troubled by the uncritical enthusiasm shown by the general public, individual physicians and American medical schools in promoting religious activities as part of medical treatment. The authors feel there is very little scientific evidence to show religious activities promote good health. Their argument is summarized here:

1. Is there evidence of a link between religion and health?

Yes. Some studies have shown regular church attendance, listening to religious television programs, praying, and reading the Bible may be associated with improved health. But the authors believe the evidence is generally weak and unconvincing, since most studies are poorly conducted. A prospective double blind trial would be most difficult to conduct.

2. *Should physicians recommend religious activity as a way of providing comfort?*

    The authors quote a study that says: "The primary task of the physician is to cure sometimes, to relieve often, and to comfort always." We know that many people do get comfort from religious activities. But is it ethical for a physician to prescribe religious activities to a patient without infringing on the patient's freedom of choice?

    The authors feel religious practices can be disruptive as well as healing, physicians are not trained to engage in in-depth conversations with their patients about their spiritual concerns, and the physician and the patient may not have the same religious beliefs. Therefore, it may not be a good idea for physicians to get into prescribing religious activities to their patients.

3. *Do patients want religious matters to be incorporated into their medical care?*

    Studies have shown 40 to 50 per cent of patients want physicians to attend to their spiritual needs. But these numbers do not emphasize the views of 50 to 60 per cent of the patients who think otherwise. Most of these surveys are on inpatients. This may not be relevant to office and outpatient work.

Religious Activities on Doctor's Orders – What do the readers of my newspaper column think?

"Religion is the opium of the people," said Karl Marx (1818-1883). But Marxism is almost dead and religion has survived. Does that mean religion is healthy and well and good for the people?

Yes, says one reader of my columns in the *Medicine Hat News*. She was responding to my question: should doctors prescribe religious activities for medical ailments as they prescribe antibiotics?

The lady (we shall call her Mrs. A) says: I am almost sure that healthy spiritual life is directly connected to good mental health.

And mental health is directly connected with physical health. It is proven that mental condition has direct influence on our immune system, hormonal balance, sleeping pattern and not to mention the impact it has on our social life. So yes, religion should be somehow involved in medical treatment.

Mrs. A says the zealots are exploiting religion. She was brought up in a country where religion was not popular and there were many atheists. Atheism was more attractive because some religious leaders encouraged hate among people of different nationality and religion.

"That was the reason I was always happy not to be a part of it, not to be in all the mess. My opinion now is that religion/spirituality is important if it's in the healthy dosage," says Mrs. A.

Another interesting letter came from another lady (Mrs. B): Being a "religious" person myself, I feel that faith and medical practice go hand in hand. I have a great deal of confidence in medical science but believe ultimately that God is "the great physician."

I think it is quite desirable for physicians to recommend patients seek spiritual comfort from appropriate pastors and counsellors, but not that doctors have to give it–unless they know the patient well and mutually agree to discuss spiritual matters, says Mrs. B.

Mrs. B sent me an article which says doctors are conducting a major research project at the Duke University Medical Centre and the Durham Veterans Affairs Medical Centre in Durham, N.C., to study the effects of prayer, imagery and touch on patients who are about to undergo angioplasty, a procedure that removes blockages from coronary arteries.

The article says the people in the Duke prayer group experience 50 to 100 per cent fewer side effects from cardiac procedures than those who aren't prayed for.

I also received a Christian Science view from Mrs. C. She says: Christian Scientists rely exclusively on prayer for healing. A Christian Scientist may ask for help from a Christian Science practitioner, who is one who devotes his or her full time to the practice of healing prayer. Testimonials over many years appearing in the Christian

Science weekly and monthly publications prove the efficacy of this healing practice. Mrs. C adds, "On a personal note, I had a small proof when, through prayer alone, a severely sprained ankle was healed overnight."

Mrs. C says, "Christian Scientists have great respect for dedicated doctors. However, Christian Science treatment is not combined with medical practice because the two methods are inherently incompatible."

These are interesting views. Whatever religious version we believe in, the ultimate force that creates an environment of well being is our faith. The faith may be in God, in our pastor, our doctor or any non-physician healer. If we don't believe in something, then I doubt whether it will help us.

21

Staying healthy and living longer

Are we a bunch of pill-popping pathetic hypochondriacs?

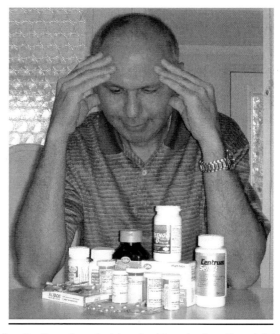

2005- Is Noorali a pill-popping pathetic hypochondriac or does he really need all these pills?

One day I was looking at some newspaper clippings on my desk. I found one from the *Globe and Mail* dated May 23, 2003. It is an article written by columnist Marcus Gee. Its title: "Stop your sniveling, you bunch of pathetic hypochondriacs."

Gee starts by saying, "People living in Canada and other rich countries today enjoy a healthier, safer life than any other generation in the whole of human history. Yet if you picked up the newspaper this week, you wouldn't know it."

Our whining and complaining goes on throughout the year. He says we have become a nation of pathetic hypochondriacs, sniveling over little hurts while people in poor countries drop dead like flies from real killers such as malaria, AIDS and tuberculosis.

Has he got a point? Are we a nation of pathetic hypochondriacs? Do we spend too many precious health-care dollars worrying about too many little things or self-inflicted illnesses?

This depends on how you perceive your health. How you feel about yourself, about your environment and what life has to offer you. If you feel you are healthy then you must be happy with yourself and what life has to offer. If you feel unwell all the time then there is something wrong somewhere.

The important thing about longevity and staying healthy is to make good choices in life and reduce the risk factors which can be genetic, environmental or lifestyle habits.

Many factors have contributed to our longevity – improvement in nutrition, public hygiene, and discovery of antibiotics, introduction of immunization programs, newer and better methods of understanding, diagnosing and treating many illnesses. Now we seem to take life for granted, especially in the industrialized and affluent countries we live in. Very few people die of infection or malnutrition. But we are still not happy. There is always something missing in our life.

Is it greed? Or are we mentally and physically weak and unhappy? We have to be mentally and physically happy to be satisfied with ourselves and our environment. Then, we may not have much to snivel about.

Our physical health depends on many things. We are healthy if we are maintaining a healthy weight, eating right, staying physically active, not smoking, controlling our blood pressure and cholesterol levels and, if diabetic, maintaining a normal blood sugar level.

The World Health Organization says in the most industrialized countries at least one-third of all disease burden is caused by:

1. tobacco
2. alcohol
3. high blood pressure
4. high cholesterol level and
5. obesity

If we want to stay healthy and live longer we need to tackle these problems.

Maintaining good weight is important. We know being overweight increases the risk of heart disease, diabetes, high blood pressure and cancer. The battle against obesity is going to be difficult just like the battle against smoking which goes on and on. There is so much good food around us it is hard not to eat and overeat.

But how does one know if a person is of normal weight?

In 2003, the *Canadian Medical Association Journal* (CMAJ) published the *Canadian Guidelines for Body Weight Classification in Adults* which updates the weight classification system that had been in use since 1988.

The authors of the article say although the guidelines are helpful, the absence of concrete answers to relevant clinical scenarios weakens their practical application, and they should be applied with caution. After all they are only guidelines. These guidelines should be used in conjunction with clinical findings.

The body weight classification depends on the body mass index (BMI) – kg/m². There are many sites on the Internet where we can enter our height and weight and our BMI will be calculated for us.

We are considered *underweight* if our BMI is lower than 18.5 kg/m². This could be a marker of malnutrition or may identify people with eating disorders.

If our BMI is between 18.5 and 24.9 kg/m² then this is considered *normal* and good weight for most people.

Overweight is defined as a BMI between 25 and 30 kg/m². This is associated with increased health risks and may lead to health problems in some people. The authors say many factors beyond BMI influence health risk, such as body fat distribution, physical activity, diet and genetic background.

Obesity is defined as an excessive accumulation of body fat. A BMI of over 30 is considered to be obese. These individuals have increased risk of health problems.

Waist circumference is also important. Healthy waist circumference in a male should be less than 102 cm and for females less than 88 cm.

If we can take care of obesity then in most instances it will take care of high blood pressure, high cholesterol level and diabetes.

The battle against smoking and excess use of alcohol is as difficult as it is against obesity. The addiction is hard to get rid of. Smokers and drinkers know the stuff is not good for them, but for whatever reason they continue to be slaves. Illnesses from these addictions destroy our health and drain our health-care system of precious dollars which can be put to better use.

It is no secret tobacco use is the leading cause of preventable illness, disability and death in the Western world. Smokers have two to four times the risk of heart attack and sudden death from coronary artery disease than non-smokers. Smoking around children can negatively impact their health. Smoking during pregnancy is associated with low birth weight and health problems in infancy and later on. Exposure to second-hand smoke can increase non-smokers' likelihood of developing asthma, heart disease and lung cancer.

There are some benefits to alcohol use if used in moderation, but definition of moderation varies according to one's tolerance level. Physicians are therefore reluctant to encourage or promote alcohol as a panacea for major health problems. *What is bad about alcohol?*

- Alcohol causes fetal alcohol syndrome in newborns
- Causes cirrhosis of liver, liver failure and pancreatitis
- Causes gastritis and bleeding
- Causes cancer of the esophagus, breast and other cancers
- Is very heavy in useless calories

What is ugly about alcohol?

- Alcoholism is considered a disease
- It is a compulsive addictive behavior
- It is a drug with complex behavioral effects
- It causes traffic- or work-related injuries
- It is a major cause of death and disability
- It destroys a person's personal life, family life and capacity to earn a decent living

If we want to stay healthy and not be pathetic hypochondriacs then we have to try and stay mentally and physically fit. It's not always easy to do but with determination and some sacrifice it can be done. Here is a 10-point plan to be healthy, happy and live a long life:

1. Be an optimist but have plan B ready if things don't work out.
2. Approach life with a sense of humour – there is always a funny side to any situation.
3. Make good choices in life. Give up on things that are stressful.
4. Exercise at least 30 minutes a day, three to five days a week. You can do more. Every movement you make helps keep your muscles trim, melt some fat, and make you feel better.
5. Do things which challenge your brain regularly. "Anyone who stops learning is old, whether at 20 or 80. Anyone who keeps learning stays young. The greatest thing in life is to keep your mind young." – Henry Ford (1863-1947).
6. Have a diet which keeps you lean. As somebody said, if you wish to grow thinner then diminish your dinner. It was in the 1930s that scientists showed underfed rodents lived up to 40 per cent longer than their well-fed counterparts.
7. Do not smoke. The reasons should be obvious to most people who are in touch with reality. For others, there is no hope. They

like to learn lessons the hard way.
8. Be involved in the community.
9. Do not speed and always wear a seatbelt. Motor-vehicle collisions and other types of accidents kill and disable many of our young people. Drive carefully, and do not drink and drive.
10. Cut your consumption of alcohol. Alcohol is a calorie-loaded drink with no nutritional value.

It is estimated if we live up to 80, then the last 10 years of our life will be spent fighting some sort of disease or disability. This burden may be reduced if we take care of our health during our better days.

Life well spent is long.

~ Leonardo Da Vinci (1452-1519)

22

※

Getting old with flatulence

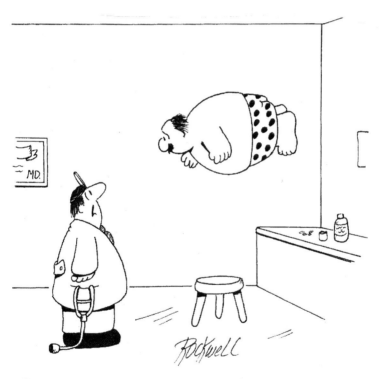

"I'm not sure what you've got, but whatever it is, it's full-blown."

NOVEMBER 1999 STITCHES

Dr. Noorali Bharwani

A question past through the ages
And pondered by many, including the sages
Is it better to hold the fart and feel the pain?
Or let the fart and feel the shame!

The above quote was sent to me by a friend. He is a banker and probably thinks that farting in his office would be shameful.

Bloating and flatulence is a significant problem in society. Almost all my patients complain of gas. My mother complains about it all the time. I am not immune to the problem. So let me ask you a question: Do you think it is shameful to "cut the cheese," or pass flatus, flatulence, wind, gas or fart–whatever you want to call it–in an environment you inhabit day and night?

After all, releasing gas is a normal and important physiological process. From birth to death, the production of gastrointestinal gas continues unhindered. It is important the product be released from our system.

"Have you passed any gas today?" is one of the first questions I ask my post-op patients, after "How are you? Did you sleep well? Do you have any pain?"

Usually the patient would say, "Yes, doctor, I burped!"

"No, did you fart today?" I would clarify in response.

Fart, or its equivalent word in different language, is the word easily understood by all living human beings irrespective of their age, sex (although females would hesitate to use the word), education or level of intelligence. Quite often though, we are afraid to use the word in public, fearing the mere mention of the word "fart" would make people smell something foul! Sorry, Dr. Pavlov!

Those who have had children will never forget the countless times we have had to wait for the baby to burp or pass flatus before he or she (I mean the baby) would finish the bottle. The release of gas had dual effect–some relief for the infant and great relief for the parent.

Do you know 97 per cent of Canadians say they suffer from intestinal gas, and about 15 per cent say they have cancelled a date or

100

a meeting because of it?

It does not matter whether you are a king or a queen, a prince or a princess, rich or poor – we all have to fart. Unfortunately, and quite often, the desire to release gas is not always at a socially convenient place.

Imagine the Queen taking a walk with Prince Phillip in the gardens of Buckingham Palace or one of the many castles and palaces she owns. Suddenly, she has a desire to release a royal fart. She looks over her shoulders to make sure nobody is behind her, especially Prince Phillip – before releasing a noisy fart.

But the important question is: Who could be following her?

Not the British public who are too pre-occupied with their own daily bowel routine.

Maybe Tony Blair, still trying to convince her about Saddam's weapons of mass destruction.

Maybe Prince Charles, looking for an excuse to plan a coup? How long can he wait to claim the throne? Maybe one unpleasant gaseous relief from the Queen would give him enough ammunition to take over the throne.

Maybe there is a paparazzo hiding behind the trees with the world's most powerful telephoto camera lens (which can pick up gas waves) accompanied by the most sophisticated sound detecting system.

What about Saddam Hussein's dilemma in that six by eight feet spider hole? For eight months he was hiding in that tiny place with little ventilation and a small fan. Once a very powerful man, he was stuck in a hole smelling his own body odour and release of intestinal gas. Did he have any gas masks with him? None that I saw on TV. He must have really missed his opulent palaces where he could fart without killing himself.

What about the astronauts who stay in space capsules and laboratories for days and months? Do they go for a walk in space to release the gas?

Some politicians are not afraid to use the word fart. For example, President Lyndon B. Johnson (1908-1973), a Democrat, said of his

Republican rival Gerald Ford, "So dumb he can't fart and chew gum at the same time." Of course, Gerald Ford went on to become president of the United States. But still he couldn't fart and chew gum at the same time.

What about Canadian politicians? Like other politicians around the world they blow a lot of gas verbally. What do they do when they have to release gas during question period, especially if you are a cabinet minister or prime minister under attack from the opposition?

Gas and bloating embrace three unrelated phenomena. Farting is a physiological phenomenon due to the production of gas by colonic bacteria. Excessive belching or burping is associated with aerophagia (air swallowing). The mechanism of bloating is obscure.

Usually, a fart consists of odourless gas–carbon dioxide and hydrogen–produced by bacterial action on carbohydrates and the proteins in the food we eat. There is methane and swallowed nitrogen as well. These four gases make up 99 per cent of colonic gas.

The remaining component consists of trace gases that compensate for their small quantities by their strong odours. Smelly gases include hydrogen sulfide, ammonia, indole and volatile fatty acids.

According to a textbook of gastroenterology, an average person on a normal diet emits about one litre of gas per day. On average we pass gas 13.6 times per day although there is a great variation from person to person, from time to time, depending on what you eat and how much air you swallow.

Patients with lactose intolerance and irritable bowel syndrome may have excess gas. You can reduce gas by eliminating certain foods (peas, beans, cauliflower, certain grain products and carbohydrates) from your diet. But most of the time there is only one way to get rid of gas–look over your shoulder and let it go!

Of course, that is not easy. Can you imagine what would happen in a concert hall, in a plane or in a meeting room full of politicians and bureaucrats? There is a social taboo associated with the use of the word "fart" and the release of gas in public. Actors such as Jim Carrey in *Dumb and Dumber* and Eddie Murphy's family dinner explosions in *The Nutty Professor*, have done their bit for humans like us to release as much gas as possible in public without feeling embarrassed. In my humble way, I feel by writing this article, I have made a small contribution in further emancipation of our mind and body.

Finally, imagine Prince Charles' frustration when he could not publicly express his love for his lover Camilla Parker-Bowles. He must have said:

> *Love is the fart*
> *Of every heart:*
> *It pains a man when 'tis kept close,*
> *And others doth offend, when 'tis let loose.*

~ with apologies to Sir John Suckling (1609-1642)

23

Jamaica and evidence-based medicine

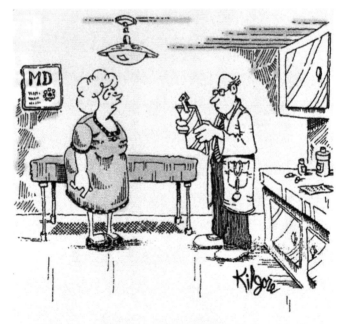

"All this medical progress I've read about and you tell me it's just a headache … ?"

From Stitches January, 2005

You see a doctor for a medical problem. He advises you to follow certain treatment. Do you ever ask him: Doctor, is there any scientific evidence to show this treatment works?

Most of us trust our doctor and are too polite to ask him such a question. Instead we rely on our neighbours, friends and families to give us a second and a third opinion.

Those who are computer literate surf the Internet. But you know what happens there – there are thousands of references to search for an answer.

What do doctors do when they are looking for best evidence in their practice?

Doctors go back to their text books, read medical journals, talk to their colleagues, have case conferences in the hospital or attend medical meetings at exotic places.

In October 2003 I went to Montego Bay, Jamaica, with my associate, Dr. Wojciech Brzezinski, to attend a two-day conference on evidence-based medicine in gastroenterology.

It was a very interesting conference. The location was beautiful, an ideal environment to learn something. The warm ocean breeze, carrying important scientific knowledge, penetrates your brain without difficulty.

There were experts from Europe, Canada and Jamaica. The main discussion was on the problems of the esophagus and stomach.

As we know, medicine is an imperfect science. Quite often the practice of medicine is more an art than science. The discussion at the Jamaican conference again confirmed that.

Only about 10 to 20 per cent of what we do in medicine is evidence based. That means it is scientifically proven. The rest is based on what each one of us think is correct, what we think is best for a particular patient that is economical and safe.

The advantage of evidence-based medicine is that it helps optimize patient care and minimize variation in best practice.

The problem is that in most cases there is not enough evidence available. Clinical decision making is a very complex process because no two patients respond to a treatment in exactly the same manner. Therefore, evidence-based medicine in clinical practice is quite often not relevant.

But in spite of imperfections in medical practice, we continue to treat hundreds and thousands of patients each day. Most of them do well and respond to treatment.

Some get better just by talking to a sympathetic doctor.

Some get better by taking an aspirin and going to bed.

Some get better by doing nothing, maybe a shot of brandy. Or Jamaican style – don't worry, be happy.

Some get better by following the principles of ELMOSS – exercise, laughter, meditation, organic/healthy food, stress relief and by giving up smoking.

Eventually most people do get better. Time is a good healer unless you are suffering from an incurable disease.

Medicine is not a rocket science. You have to know the human anatomy, physiology, pharmacology and pathology. Then you learn about medicine, surgery, gynecology, obstetrics, ophthalmology, ear, nose and throat surgery. Then you have to put all this knowledge together and pass a few exams. Then you can call yourself a doctor of medicine and surgery!

Isn't that easy? It just takes 10 to 15 years of your life. Then you start a practice and find out that only 20 per cent of what you practice is based on pure science. But you can say, I have been to Jamaica!

Seriously, next time you are sick.................see your doctor first!

Who shall decide when doctors disagree?
~ Alexander Pope (1688-1744)

24

Quick Q & A with the *Medical Post*

November 19, 2002

What is your least favourite medical procedure that you regularly perform?
Not a medical procedure but part of it: filling out insurance forms.

What book are you reading?
Jacalyn Duffin's *History of Medicine: A Scandalously Short Introduction.*

What illness do you most fear getting?
Hepatitis or AIDS.

What do you think is the most exciting field of science at the moment?
Medical genetics.

What is the least enjoyable job you've ever had?
Working as a stock boy at a supermarket in London, England, while waiting for my General Medical Council registration.

What do you do when you need to clear your mind?
Watch a comedy show, go on a treadmill or meditate.

What is the best piece of advice you've ever been given?
"Be an optimist but have plan B ready."

What vice do you have that you hide from patients?
My short fuse – if that is a vice!

What is your biggest extravagance?
My office building.

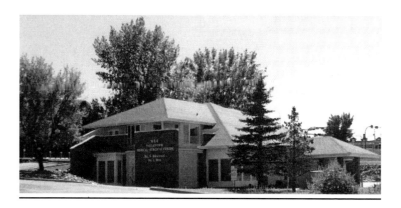

What talent do you envy in others?
Singing.

What is your favourite meal?
My wife's vegetable soup.

What do you say to someone who says doctors have it made?
Try going through a medical school and residency program, then come and talk to me.

What do you think is the greatest political danger to the medical profession?
Politicians do not understand that medicine is an imperfect science with many promises and expectations which cannot be satisfactorily delivered without adequate funding, manpower, equipment and infrastructure.

What's your junk-food weakness?
Chocolate chip peanut butter cookies from Tim Horton's! Our hospital Tim Horton's is out of bounds for me, so I am going through withdrawal symptoms.

25

A doctor's prayer

I would like to share this prayer with the readers of my book. This was given to me by Sister Alfrieda, a very wonderful and caring person. I have the prayer posted on the wall in every examination room in my office.

As I care for my patients today,

Be there with me O Lord I pray.

Let me speak kind words that mean so much

And in my hands place your healing touch.

Let your love shine through all that I do,

So those in need may hear and feel you.

Amen.

26

What others say...
Just a few examples:

From an author/editor: Noorali, you have a charm about your writing so I have little doubt you'll be successful.

From an author: I like your style, humour, down-to-earth easy approachableness. You are at your best when you relate autobiographical material.

From psychologist A: You have that genuine personal approach which gives the material its authenticity, and which makes it so readable.

From psychologist B: I have enjoyed your regular column in the *Medicine Hat News* but never as much as the one describing your recent illness. You have wonderful sense of humour and I believe that your honesty is admirable. Many professionals would "retreat" or try to be private in times of difficulties. Good job!

From a health administrator: I think you do a wonderful job of putting a personal face on religious and historical issues. Yours is a voice of reason, humanity and humour in this sometimes perplexing world. Please keep up the good work (and words) in your columns.

Letter to editor, the Medicine Hat News: I am always looking forward to What's Up Doc?–Dr. Bharwani's column on health. It offers such good advice and is easily understood. He has great concern about the well-being of people. Thank you Dr. Bharwani.

From a cousin: I read your columns with great interest and have benefited a lot from the information and the advice that you give. ***From a nursing instructor:*** Dr. Bharwani, I enjoy your columns. I often post them on my door at the college for my nursing students to read.

From a physician colleague: I enjoyed your most recent column. It was full of interesting information and practical advice. I read or scan most of your columns. They are filled with valuable information and health advice for the public. This is a wonderful service you perform. Thanks! Keep up the great work!!

27

※

A recipe for success

Hard work

+

Perseverance

+

Good friends

+

A devoted family

=

Success

28

Last page prescription

Don't worry, be happy and laugh a lot!

Laughter is the closest thing to the grace of God.
~ Karl Bath (1886-1968)

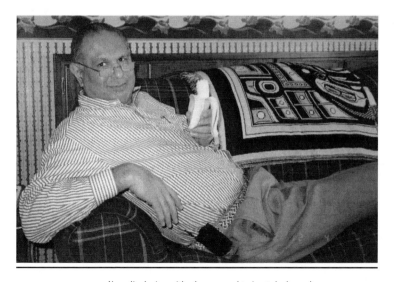

2002 – Noorali relaxing with a banana and trying to be happy!

So many gods, so many creeds,
So many paths that wind and wind,
While just the art of being kind
Is all the sad world needs.

~ Ella Wheeler Wilcox (1855-1919)

An intellectual is a man who takes more words than necessary to tell more than he knows.

~ Dwight Eisenhower (1890-1969)

ISBN 141209156-X